Journey Through Brain Trauma

Journey Through
BRAIN TRAUMA

A Mother's Story
of Her Daughter's Recovery

⊚

LOUISE RAY MORNINGSTAR

with ALEXIA DORSZYNSKI

TAYLOR PUBLISHING COMPANY, DALLAS, TEXAS

Names of certain individuals in this book have been
changed to protect privacy.

Published by Taylor Publishing Company
1550 West Mockingbird Lane
Dallas, Texas 75235

Book design by Mark McGarry
Set in Aldus

Library of Congress Cataloging-in-Publication Data
Morningstar, Louise Ray. Journey through brain trauma :
a mother's story of her daughter's recovery / Louise Ray Morningstar,
with Alexia Dorszynski.
p. cm.
ISBN 0–87833–988–4
1. Morningstar, Misti—Health. 2. Brain damage—patients—United
States—Biography. I. Dorszynski, Alexia. II. Title.
RC387.5.M67   1998   362.1′98928′0092—dc21
[B]   98–11005
CIP

Printed in the United States of America
10 9 8 7 6 5 4 3 2 1

To my children, Cork, Chuck, and Misti

Laugh often,
love children,
believe in miracles,
appreciate beauty,
find the best in others,
strive to make the world a better place,
and know that touching someone else's life in a
positive way is life's greatest success

Contents

Acknowledgments

I have many people to thank, wonderful people who have helped me, many who have shared my journey. My heartfelt thanks goes to God, my wonderful husband and family, doctors, colleagues, and friends of whom there are many too many to name individually. May each of them know that without their support Misti and I could not have survived our journey. Thanks, too, to those who have encouraged me to share my experience in the hope that it may help others.

My deepest gratitude to Alexia Dorszynski, whose help in writing this book has been invaluable, and to Faith Hamlin, my agent, who is responsible for helping it find a good home.

Prologue

Despite the bone-chilling cold, seventeen-year-old Misti Morningstar is determined to carry out the plans she and her companion Carol have outlined for the day—a shopping expedition to the Lake Forest Mall not far from Washington, D.C. On this cold February morning, Misti drives the little blue Subaru, with Carol, her boyfriend's aunt, acting as navigator. Waiting second in line for the red light at the intersection of Midcounty Highway and Goshen Road to turn green, Misti remarks that the Subaru's heater has finally begun to puff out some heat.

Approaching the crossroad, truck driver Richard Edward Winslow glances down at the hand-written directions to the job site where he is scheduled to deliver the thirty-two tons of concrete pipe loaded on the flat bed pulled by his red Mack tractor. He is preoccupied by the directions in his hand and doesn't notice that the green light at the intersection has slipped through yellow and turned red or that the cross traffic has started to move. He looks up only as he hears the sound of metal striking metal and feels the slight jolt of his truck. His braking reaction comes too late. The eighteen-wheeler he drives has run over the little car, smashing it as easily as if it were a toy in the path of some great giant.

The momentum of the loaded truck keeps it from stopping until it has edged over the embankment on the other side of the road. Tons of concrete piping roll in all directions, some of it coming to rest beside the crumpled blue car.

At 11:05 A.M. the Montgomery County police receive a call reporting the accident. Police and ambulances arrive, sirens screaming, and a crowd soon gathers. The air is filled with shouts of "Over here," "Someone help," "Oh, my God," and "How many people are in there?" An authoritative voice commands, "Stand back," and then speaks into a two-way radio. "Call for a copter."

Richard Winslow stands by the side of the road, unharmed except for his shock. The thirty-nine-year-old stammers to a uniformed policeman, "I never saw the intersection."

1

A medi-vac helicopter from Suburban Hospital in nearby Bethesda arrives. At the same time, the regular paramedics, who have been trained to rescue crash victims in the least traumatic way, are working feverishly to remove the woman trapped in the passenger side of the car. After a few minutes, they are able to lift her out. She is covered with blood. Medics strap her to a backboard to prevent possible spinal injury and place her in an ambulance, which roars away en route to the Shock Trauma Unit at Suburban Medical Center in Bethesda.

Meanwhile, work continues at the accident scene. The little blue car has been crushed like a cardboard box, and somewhere, buried beneath the twisted metal of car and truck, is the car's driver. As special tools cut away the mangled car, the paramedics locate a small, rag-doll body, still as death. Slowly, painstakingly, they cut the girl from the tangle of debris. She is covered with so much blood and dirt that it is impossible to tell the color of her long hair. The medic who has arrived in the copter assesses the scene quickly, knowing that seconds count. Because blood is still flowing from the girl's injuries, he knows that she is still alive, but it is imperative to stop the blood loss if she is to have even a small chance of survival. Acting instinctively, he quickly begins to cut the clothing from the girl's upper body, exposing her upper torso to the icy wind in hopes of slowing her circulation, and, he hopes, easing the loss of blood from her head injuries. One of the other paramedics wraps a warm blanket around her lower body to try to counteract the effects of shock. Then she is loaded into the copter.

The helicopter lifts off the ground, arriving only minutes later at Suburban Medical Center. Alerted by radio, nurses await the copter's arrival at the circular pad in front of the medical facility and quickly take charge.

The girl's still, almost lifeless body is wheeled into an operating room, where doctors have been standing by. Here the remainder of her clothing is cut away. The gold jewelry she is wearing is placed in a plastic bag marked "personal," her contact lenses are removed, and a plastic hospital bracelet with the name "Jane Doe" is clasped around her limp wrist.

Time is of the essence now and the medical team works quickly, quietly, urgently. The doctors note that the girl is unconscious, with labored, shallow breathing; her neck is in a Philadelphia collar to guard against possible injury, and an X-ray is taken to make sure that she has suffered no injury to her neck or spine. As soon as the spinal X-ray is complete, a tube is inserted into her throat and oxygen is administered. The emergency team, noting that the paramedics had been unable to get an IV going, begin looking for usable veins. Chest X-rays are taken, as is a CT (computer tomography) scan of the head. This last test, which provides multiple cross-section views of the brain, like carrot coins or pieces of sausage, is probably the most vital—and the most informative—because it reveals that there have been contusions and bruising to the right frontal and left parietal lobes of the brain, with swelling of the cerebrum. The neurosurgeon who is part of the trauma team places an intracranial monitor in the girl's head to keep track of the brain's swelling and any resultant pressure. The girl's abdomen is washed, revealing bleeding; an exploratory laparotomy (an abdominal incision) is performed, showing that the blood is coming from a ruptured ovary, which is immediately oversewn. Directly thereafter, she is taken to the Shock Trauma Unit, where she is put on a ventilator. As the gurney leaves the operating room, one of the nurses whispers, with much love, "She is in God's hands now."

When brain trauma occurs, the first priority is to monitor the damage and stabilize the patient's overall condition. If damage to the brain is too severe, the patient may not survive at all. With enough damage to the brain, the patient may survive the trauma but never recover consciousness. In accidents such as Misti's, the damage to the brain comes not only from the impact of the skull against a steering wheel, car door, or windshield, but also from the soft tissue of the brain colliding with the hard tissue of skull bone at the front of the head and then slamming backward toward the rear of the skull—action that is likely to result in the bruising of the delicate, nerve-laden brain tissue. Beyond the danger of immediate trauma is that of swelling in the small, contained space of the skull. Swelling of the injured brain can itself cause more trauma as nerves are compressed against brain tissue or bone.

The frontal lobes of the brain plan for the future, control movement, and produce speech; the parietal lobes receive and process data from the senses. Misti's CT confirms that both have suffered trauma. The occipital lobes, which specialize in vision, and the temporal lobes, which hear and interpret music and language, have also received some damage. Only time will tell if the amygdala, which is buried deep in the center of the brain and generates emotions from perceptions and thoughts, or the nearby hippocampus, which has the job of consolidating recently acquired information, somehow turning short-term memory into long-term, will be spared, or whether swelling from the bruising will cause further damage.

For now, what's clear is that the life of Misti Morningstar, an honors student planning a career in medicine, a beloved daughter and younger sister, a dancer, a roommate, and a girlfriend, has been sharply altered. The real question just now is whether she will be able to survive this devastating brain trauma at all.

One

The greatest journey of my life began on a sunny day in February 1988. My husband Harry and I were enjoying an unhurried, truly relaxing vacation with friends in a quiet resort about two miles from the capital city of St. John in the Virgin Islands. There the smiling sun and cooling trade winds worked hand in hand to make nearly every day picture perfect.

The trip marked both an end and a new beginning. After nearly thirty-five years of marriage and partnership in two successful family businesses in our hometown of Waynesboro, Pennsylvania, Harry and I had decided that we were ready to go in a new direction. Our seventeen-year-old daughter Misti was attending boarding school and would soon be ready for college, and our sons Chuck and Cork were well-launched in the world, with families of their own. In the last several months, we had formally sold Waynesboro Decorating and The Furniture Market to our sons, freeing Harry to explore new business ventures and take more of the fishing and hunting trips he loved. And I now had more time to spend with my friends, grandchildren, and aging parents. Of course, I would still be involved in some decorating projects, and Harry and I would both make ourselves available to help when and if the boys asked, but for now we were enjoying our hard-earned holiday in the sun.

On that last innocent day, Harry and I had had a leisurely lunch at the marina in Dickenson Bay, drinking iced tea as we discussed how lucky we were. Neither of us came from wealthy or influential families, but hard work and careful planning had allowed us to prosper. Now, we were enjoying the good life, experiencing things we would not have imagined as children. We could not have anticipated at the time that we had just had the last carefree conversation we would have for five years.

When we arrived back at the hotel shortly after six, we were told that our son had called, and he would call again every hour on the hour until he reached us. Since the island's antiquated phone system would not allow us to make a call to the States very easily, we settled down to wait. Our friend Sue said, "If you need us, just call," and then she and her husband Ronnie headed discreetly to their room. I reflected that the news was most likely that the condition of my father, who was in the late stages of Alzheimer's disease, had gotten worse. The phone rang a few minutes later, and with that, our family nightmare began.

On the phone was Chuck, the younger of our two sons, though I could barely recognize his voice; he was terribly upset, crying, and he asked to speak to his dad. Harry took the phone and began to listen. A look of horror came over his face, the color drained from his newly tanned cheeks, and his heart began to beat so hard that I could see it through the thin blue knit shirt he wore. When he dropped the earpiece of the phone back onto the receiver and looked at me, I was sure that the bad news concerned his mother, now in her eighties. Instead, his lips shaped the words, "Misti—it's Misti—she's been in an accident." He began to explain what Chuck had told him, but I could not take it in. I heard my own voice screaming: "No, no!" When Sue and Ronnie ran in, Harry was slumped in disbelief on the bed; one look told them that something terrible had happened.

I was aware of Sue leaving the room, then I felt my stomach churning and had to run into the bathroom, where I was violently ill. Though Chuck had really given us no details, just that Misti was hurt, it was clear that we should do something quickly—get to Misti, wherever she was. But for that stunned moment, time seemed to have stopped. Then Sue reappeared, briskly but kindly issuing commands: "Get your toothbrushes and pills." We had only twenty minutes before a plane departing for the States was to leave, and the next one would not leave until the following night.

The airport was not crowded; at the end of the runway sat a 727, engines running and ready for takeoff. As Sue gave me a hug, I asked

5

her to pray, adding, "Please pray that if Misti cannot get better, she dies rather than suffer." I looked at Harry, and for the first time in our many years together, I saw tears in his eyes. As I sat down, I began to realize what I had just said, and I asked myself whether I could possibly have meant it; after all, Misti was our miracle baby, the much longed-for daughter we'd adopted and welcomed into our family as an infant and had loved and cared for ever since.

There were many empty seats aboard the plane. A stewardess sat down with us, offering to get brandy as soon as the plane took off; clearly, someone had let her know our situation. Then the engines roared, and I felt the familiar pressure and lift of takeoff. But this trip would not be like the others whose pictures filled the family albums— the sales incentive trips to Hawaii or Hong Kong sponsored by our suppliers, which were always happy occasions for relaxing and celebrating business success. This time, I realized with a shock, we did not even know where the plane would land. But the important thing was, it would put us closer to Misti.

As the plane flew northward, I found myself thinking about the family. Harry, Jr.—Cork, to all who knew him—was our oldest. He had been just eleven years old when we asked him what he thought of having a baby sister. Even at that age, he had been very fastidious, and he was concerned that a baby might cause the house to smell. After a long family discussion, both he and his eight-year-old brother Ora Ray, who was nicknamed Chuck, agreed that it might be a good idea to take a baby who needed a home to be part of our family.

Although Harry and I both wanted a larger family, I had miscarried a number of times between the boys' births and a number of times after Chuck's birth as well. The idea of adopting a baby girl became a real family campaign, and in two years' time, the Morningstars were blessed with a lovely baby girl with big brown eyes. Cork soon became the proud big brother, all reservations about baby smells long gone. And Chuck had always adored and spoiled and worried over Misti; that was undoubtedly why he had sounded so very upset on the telephone. After all, Chuck would become distraught if Misti so much as skinned her knee, so perhaps he had overreacted and Misti was only a little bit hurt—though of course he had been right to let us know about the accident and tell us to come home.

When the pilot's voice came over the loudspeaker and announced that we would be arriving at JKF International in a few minutes' time, I realized that this was the first we had heard of our destination. Harry and I would have to have faith that we would somehow be able to find out exactly where Misti was and how to get there. Sure enough, at the gate, we saw a man carrying a sign that read "MORNINGSTAR." He led us to a door where a gentleman in a tux and heavy overcoat was waiting near a large black limousine. In our haste to leave St. John, we had not given any thought to the weather we might encounter. We were dressed in summer clothes and sandals, and the temperature in New York was a frigid five degrees. Fortunately, the limo had already been warmed up. As we rushed away, the driver explained that he had been hired to drive us from the airport to Suburban Hospital in Bethesda, and since he was unfamiliar with the area, he would be contacting the hospital by car phone when we were closer. The staff at the hospital would be able to give him directions, and we would also be able to get a report on Misti's condition.

On the drive from New York City to Bethesda, Harry kept telling me that he was sure everything was going to be fine, that in all likelihood, Misti had had only a minor accident. After all, he reminded me, if any of our children was likely to be hurt in an accident, it would have been daredevil Chuck—whose early driving career had included more than one trip to the emergency room and whose grandfather had once suggested that it would be more efficient to attach the fenders of his car with zippers than with bolts. No, it certainly wouldn't be Misti, who was a supercautious and conscientious driver. In any case, said Harry, I'm sure that nothing terrible has happened and that the boys are handling it well.

Several hours later, the limo driver told us that he had called the hospital for directions and had also gotten good news for us: Our daughter was still alive. Harry and I just looked at each other, stunned. The driver's words had punctured our previous mood of hopeful levity. Now we just wanted to get to Misti as quickly as possible.

When we arrived at the door of the hospital, we found the area completely deserted except for two nurses waiting outside—for us. One nurse stayed with Harry, who had just realized that our supply of travelers' checks was still in St. John and was searching his pockets for money to pay the limousine driver. The other nurse took me gently by the arm and whispered urgently, "Hurry, she is still alive." We stumbled through the Emergency Room entrance, into an elevator, and down a long, barely lit hallway, with Harry running behind to catch up with us. It was now two in the morning, and everything was eerily quiet.

In the waiting room outside the Shock Trauma Unit were Chuck and Cork, my brother and his wife, and Misti's boyfriend, Max, along with his parents and his brother. Though Chuck and Cork had been sleeping, both jumped up the second we entered the room. For a few minutes massive confusion reigned, as Chuck and Cork both talked at once. Cork told us how he had heard about the accident, driven down to Bethesda, and called friends and relatives until he was able to find out where we were, while Chuck kept blurting out, "Mom, she's really hurt, Misti's really hurt."

Moments later a nurse from the Shock Trauma Unit (STU) came to take us to see Misti. Outside the entrance to the STU a phone hangs on the wall; as we would come to know so well, anyone entering the unit—doctors, nurses, technicians, and healthcare workers, as well as family and clergy—had to call first to gain admittance to the restricted area beyond the double doors.

This was clearly a place of grimness, anxiety, and crisis. It carried the unmistakable smell of antiseptic and the beeping technology that has become synonymous with modern healthcare. As we were led past several glass-enclosed rooms, I concentrated on trying to ignore the sense that death was hovering at each door. Finally, we were at the entrance to Misti's room. Taking a deep breath and clinging to each other for comfort, Harry and I went in.

At first I could barely see Misti for all the machines surrounding her. Could this still figure be our healthy, lively, daughter, the one-time ballerina whose current dream was to go to medical school, the young woman on the brink of college, of adulthood? It took a minute for the scene to start making sense to me. The room was silent, except for the machines that were keeping Misti alive. With every breath she took, a large accordion-like canister went up and down. Every heartbeat was registered by a beep and a bright light on a screen. She seemed to be connected to dozens of tubes running from her nose, her mouth, and both arms. She was nearly nude, and a large incision ran from her breast bone to the bottom of her abdomen. Her arms were motionless, and I noticed that both her wrists had deep gashes that had been stitched up. Later, when I questioned the nurse about them, she explained that in the rush to save Misti's life, the ER crew had had to cut quickly to gain access to her veins.

Her head was covered with bandages, and there were tubes and lines coming from those bandages as well. Misti's beautiful face was unmarked, her head bent ever so slightly toward her left shoulder. Besides the bandages on her head and the incisions, the only marks to indicate there had been an accident were a few scratches on her left hand. She looked so fragile that I was almost afraid to touch her, but motherly instinct made me take her hand and bend down to kiss it.

Although Harry and I had dozens of questions, we had to wait until morning for answers. The accident and the emergency brain surgery had taken place more than twelve hours before, and although Misti's condition was extremely critical, it was also stable for the moment. Unless there were a change in Misti's condition before then, the nurses explained, the doctors would talk to us after morning rounds. "Will she live?" I blurted out, afraid of the answer and yet needing to know. The nurses could tell us very little, but one of them answered kindly, "Every hour she lives gives her a better chance." We were to hear various versions of this statement many times in the next several weeks, and we had to cling to the hope it represented.

After only a few short minutes with Misti—in the STU, visits are generally very short—we were ushered back into the waiting room. There Max, the handsome seventeen-year-old Misti had been dating for months, stood by looking extremely serious, frightened, and overwhelmed. Max's parents, Brenda and Anthony, explained that the hospital's social worker had reached Max when Carol was brought into the hospital and identified, and that Max had been able to tell them Misti's name and help get word to Chuck and Cork. Although Misti had received the brunt of the accident's blow, Carol had also been hurt and was elsewhere in the hospital recovering from broken ribs.

After much discussion, Harry and I were able to persuade Cork and Chuck to go home and get some rest; in the twelve hours since Misti's surgery, her condition had not changed, and there was little that Cork or Chuck could do to be of immediate help. Max and his family stayed with us until morning. Although we all felt exhausted and helpless, we were afraid to go to sleep; if Misti's condition changed, we wanted to be there with her. In the meantime, all we could do was pray.

The rest of that night had a nightmarish quality to it. Yesterday, Misti had been healthy and happy, her biggest concerns an upcoming prom and which colleges might accept her, and Harry and I had been vacationing in the Caribbean. Now we were in a hospital waiting room, wondering whether our daughter would live or die.

As promised, the doctors arrived around 7:00 A.M. Dr. Jamshidi, the neurosurgeon, explained that Misti's brain had been bruised in the accident and that he and the other doctors had made some holes in Misti's skull to relieve the pressure from the swelling; they had also installed a monitor to keep track of the pressure within her skull. At present, she was recovering from the surgery and we could hope that the swelling in her brain would soon start to subside; as long as the swelling did not continue, as long as Misti did not remain in a coma for too long, there was a chance that she would recover. But the longer the coma went on, the greater the damage was likely to be. The neurosurgeon was accompanied by several other specialists, and they all tried to be informative and even vaguely comforting. But I grasped only that Misti's condition was very critical, that she was in a coma, and that it might be a long time before we knew whether or how much she would recover. The doctors also repeated what the nurses had told us the night before: Each hour she lived gave her a better chance. But the tone of their voices reflected the near hopelessness of Misti's condition, and fear gripped our hearts.

Two

After talking to the doctors, Harry and I realized that we were very likely to be in for a siege. At this point, I was still expecting that Misti would soon open her eyes and say, "Where am I? What happened?" like the heroine of a movie. At the same time, I was still trying to deal with the shock of it all. Misti had been fine only yesterday morning, her face was untouched, she looked as though she was sleeping. Why couldn't she just wake up?

A number of family members and friends—Harry's brother Dave and his wife Becky; his Uncle Ora and Aunt Goldie, who were like parents to him; and our friends Bonnie and Rani Carniello, and Joyce and Tom Mock—came down to be with us at various points as we kept our vigil. Harry and I barely moved from the STU's waiting room for three days. Fortunately, Uncle Ora and Aunt Goldie brought us both a change of clothes, so we were finally able to change into clothes more appropriate for winter.

Although we were still hopeful that Misti would soon emerge from the coma, it was clear that she would need us to be close by for awhile. We stayed at the hospital the first night; then Max's parents insisted that we get some sleep at their home, which was fifteen minutes away from the hospital. The second night Harry went home with them, and the third night he stayed at the hospital while I accepted their hospitality. The next day, Harry, who was used to being very active and was finding the tense waiting very difficult to endure, announced that he had to get some air. Stepping into his accustomed role of provider and protector, he then took the opportunity to find us a suite in a clean and serviceable hotel near the hospital. Since we had no idea how long we would need it, we rented the suite day by day; ultimately, we would be there for a month.

After the first few days, the stream of visitors subsided, with most people keeping in touch by telephone. Sitting alone in the waiting room outside the STU, Harry and I began to sort through the helter-skelter of our lives. Our car was in the long-term parking lot of the Philadelphia airport, our luggage and clothes were still at the hotel in St. John, and soon business concerns would be pressing upon us again. Meanwhile, we gratefully accepted the help that friends and relatives offered; it was especially helpful when people from our church volunteered to take calls and give information for us, taking the burden off Chuck and Cork and their office staff. Our pastor told us that a prayer chain for Misti's recovery had been started in our church. We also learned that prayers were being said for Misti in North Carolina, where I had cousins, in Alaska, where Harry's cousin and his family lived, and even as far away as Guyana, in Africa, where the parents of Odette Harper, Misti's roommate at Mercersburg Academy, lived.

Odette had heard the news about Misti in the world's most awful way—over the radio, with no warning. Odette had been on a trip to Washington, D.C., with Mr. Needham, a Mercersburg Academy chemistry teacher and coach, and several members of the basketball team when the van's radio blasted out the news that Misti Morningstar had been in an accident. It couldn't be her Misti, Odette had told herself, but after all, how many Misti Morningstars are there?

From Mr. Burgin, the headmaster, we learned that the Mercersburg Academy, the rigorous prep school that Misti had been attending for the past three years, had started a program of education and counseling for Misti's fellow students. Teenagers all believe they are immortal, that nothing bad can happen to them. Now Misti's schoolmates were learning about "traumatic brain injury" and the terrible vulnerability of human life.

At the STU, only immediate family members and clergy were allowed to visit the patients, and for only five minutes at a time, three times a day. As we waited to see Misti again, time crawled, and I found myself thinking about Mercersburg Academy and our search for the right school for Misti.

Misti had always been very bright—a high academic achiever as well as a talented dancer—and the local public schools were just not challenging enough for her. When it became clear that she needed more than her classes there could offer, Misti tried programs at several local private schools, before settling on Mercersburg Academy, a small, coed, mostly residential prep school thirty miles from Waynesboro. Mercersburg was a proud old school, with tough academics, a strict dress code, and a solid disciplinary tradition. Students actually "walked guard" as punishment for infractions of the rules. They came from all over the world, and despite their varied backgrounds, the kids in each class were a close-knit bunch, functioning almost like a family.

Misti had taken to Mercersburg like a duck to water. Not only had she done very well academically, she had served as the copy editor of the school's yearbook and head manager of the baseball and basketball teams. She and Odette had been roommates and fast friends for two and a half years, both planning careers in medicine and urging each other on academically. They had applied to colleges the previous fall and were now waiting to see where they'd be accepted. But here I shook my head: Misti had said for years that she wanted to go to medical school, and we'd always assumed that her talent and single-minded determination would allow her to do just that. Now I had to wonder whether Misti would survive and recover enough to graduate from Mercersburg.

◎

In a few short days, the waiting room outside the STU became home, as familiar as our house in Waynesboro. In the month Misti was in the STU, we came to know the bland wall covering, the institutional furniture, and the faded blue blinds all too well.

Every day, the routine was the same. We'd arrive at the hospital about 8:00 A.M., find out what kind of night Misti had had, and wait for those precious five-minute intervals when we were allowed to be with her. We'd call Cork and Chuck and their families after each visit, sharing what little news we had. Harry and I took turns going to the hospital cafeteria, eating food that was undoubtedly nutritious but carried the distinct flavor of anxiety. We tried to reassure each other. And we prayed.

From time to time, new faces would appear in the waiting room, each carrying the same look of shock and terror that we had had on arrival. By now we knew that there were ten beds in the STU. Sometimes all the beds were filled, sometimes not, but we never saw the comings and goings of the patients, who were transported through a different entrance. We did get to know some of the families with whom we shared our frightening vigil: the parents of the young man with a gunshot wound to the head, the parents of an honors student and class valedictorian who had been in an accident similar to Misti's, the spouses of the stroke victims. Every now and again a nurse or a doctor would come through the door and ask Mr. and Mrs. So-and-so to step outside with them. Next we would hear sobs—and know that our new friends would not be returning. Their loved one was gone. This happened as often as three times a day, and every time that door opened, my heart contracted with fear: Would they call us this time? No one ever really got good news; the best one could hope for was a patient's transfer to another medical facility of some sort.

Time passed, but Misti's coma was not like one in the movies: She did not move or recover consciousness. The doctors told us that the various probes measuring Misti's brain activity showed delta waves, which point toward deep coma, and her brain continued to swell. Now every additional hour she was unconscious meant more injury to the brain.

Three days after the accident, Max's aunt Carol was discharged from the hospital. When she stopped in to see us at the STU waiting room, she was in obvious pain. I found myself wondering whether God in his mercy had put Misti in a coma because she could not bear the pain she would otherwise be feeling.

On the weekend that followed, Cork and Chuck and their wives came down to visit with us, but there were problems getting everyone in to see Misti because the wives were not considered immediate family. Furthermore, the staff of the STU felt that it was extremely important that no one be upset around Misti, whose blood pressure and heart rate went up when she heard sounds that disturbed her; anyone who was likely to sound distressed was gently asked to leave. Everyone asked what they could do to help, but the only real answer was "Pray," and they were all doing that already.

By this time, Harry and I had read everything the hospital offered on traumatic brain injury and had begun to look for some sign that Misti's brain was beginning to heal. However, the next piece of news we got was bad: One of Misti's lungs had collapsed and needed to be reinflated. She was also suffering a number of medical complications, among them small seizures, several infections, and blood clots. Further, the accident had damaged the part of Misti's brain that regulates the metabolism, and her blood work showed that she was on the verge of diabetes. Still, following the suggestions of the hospital staff, we talked encouragingly to Misti about her recovery just as though she could understand us, and we made sure that her room was filled with photographs of friends and family members.

Larry Jones, the Mercersburg chaplain and one of Misti's favorite people, came down to visit and pray with us one day that first week. He tried hard to hold his emotions in check, but he was clearly quite pained and fearful for Misti. Later that day, Pastor Clark came down from our church in Waynesboro and anointed her with oil; in the Lutheran tradition, the gravely ill are anointed with oil as the faithful pray for their recovery—if it is God's will. Meanwhile, the doctors ordered new CT scans, which seemed to show that the swelling in the brain had begun to abate—though not enough to give any real hope. As they kept repeating, even if Misti's overall physical condition began to improve, the longer that she was in the coma, the greater the resulting brain damage.

☙

Five days after the accident, as I was trying to console members of a family who had just arrived in the waiting room, a nurse opened the door and called for the Morningstars. My heart stood still as I took the ten most terrifying steps in the world. But it was not the news we so feared. Instead, the nurse explained that Misti's hair was starting to pose a serious problem. Although the top of it had been shaved before the emergency brain surgery, the thick hair at the back and sides of her head had remained untouched, almost literally so. It was still loaded with the dried blood and debris from the accident, and the staff considered it a possible source of infection—surely the last thing Misti needed. It seemed that there was nothing to do but shave the rest of Misti's head. As the nurse spoke, I decided that I could not let this happen. When Misti came out of the coma—and suddenly, I was convinced that this would indeed happen—she would be very upset to find that I had let her head be shaved. I pleaded for a twenty-four-hour reprieve to give me time to think; the nurse gave me twelve hours. As I lay awake that night, my mind was busy, considering plan after plan. Perhaps I could take a washcloth or sponge and wash the blood out of Misti's hair strand by strand and then dress it in small braids to get it out of the way. I thought this would work. I hoped it would work. It had to work.

In the morning, two friends unexpectedly arrived from Waynesboro. They volunteered to help me deal with Misti's hair. We assembled plastic sheets, a basin, wash cloths, and a hair pick, working slowly and carefully, trying hard not to hurt Misti and making sure that she did not catch a chill. Later in the day, we had a visit from Uncle Ora, Aunt Goldie, and their minister. The minister talked and prayed with us, saying that today he had truly witnessed what could only be described as a labor of love. He then looked at Harry and me and told us to go back to the hotel and make love—his way of saying we should move on with our lives. We looked at each other and smiled, a little embarrassed. I knew that he was right and that life must go on, but it was strange to hear this particular bit of advice from a Brethren minister.

Misti's best friend from Waynesboro, Rani Carniello, came down for a day that first week, and over a snack in the cafeteria, she announced what I had already come to believe: Misti was going to get well. Rani said she knew this because her dad, who had died a few days after Christmas, was the new kid on the block up in heaven, and being the typical Italian, he was surely shaking his fist in someone's face, telling them that Misti had to survive this. Rani laughed as I commented, "Let's hope the fist is directed to St. Peter and not the big man himself."

But it seemed that Rani's father was not shaking his fist in the right face. A few days later, Misti developed pneumonia, a common and quite serious complication for coma patients, which threatened her already shaky chances for survival. But this blow was softened when we learned that the latest scans seemed to indicate that the blood clots on her brain had begun to dissolve. We redoubled our efforts, talking to Misti and playing music she might recognize, in the hope of stimulating some kind of response. Yet she continued to lie apparently lifeless—still beautiful, but now thin and pale. Why wasn't she fighting, we wondered. She had always been ready to tackle the next challenge life handed out. Why not now?

One night, some old friends from high school came down and persuaded us to take a brief break from the STU. Buoyed by the love and encouragement of these old friends, we allowed ourselves to hope that Misti would soon start to fight—only to learn when we returned to the hospital that Misti's temperature had gone up again. She had to be placed on an ice blanket in an effort to lower it. Each degree of fever not only interfered with the healing process but also made the brain damage worse.

By the middle of the week, Misti's feet and hands had begun to draw into contorted positions—what the doctors said was "decerebrate posturing." Her toes had begun to point down, shortening her Achilles' tendons in what the nurses called "foot drop." Casts were made and splints applied so that she would not be badly crippled when she finally came out of her coma.

It had now been nine days since the accident, and we had to accept that time was passing and that our lives, though very much changed, also had to go on. There was no reason for everyone to sit and wait for something to happen when changes would likely be very slow in coming. Many months previously, Harry had purchased tickets for an Elk Preservation Dinner in Harrisburg, Pennsylvania, and we now decided that he and Cork would use the tickets, staying in Harrisburg overnight. Harry had been terribly upset by the accident—a typical doting father, he would do anything for his little girl and was frustrated that he could do so little—and he needed a break from the awful hospital routine. Nonetheless, I was glad I had decided to stay; the next morning, Misti seemed to move her right hand slightly as I held it in mine. Even as my heart leapt, however, I had to acknowledge that I could well be imagining it.

Two weeks after the accident, Misti's Mercersburg roommate, Odette, received permission to leave campus and came down to Bethesda for a visit. As Odette and I walked hand in hand through the STU doors and toward Misti's room, I glanced down at our clasped hands, thinking of the song "Ebony and Ivory." After our five-minute visit with Misti, one of the nurses reminded me about the immediate-family-and-clergy-only rule. Keeping my face straight but unable to keep a smile out of my voice, I told her that Odette was Misti's sister but that they had different fathers. The nurse smiled softly, clearly recognizing that these two girls could not be closer if they really were related. They came from opposite sides of the world, but they had shared all the secrets of high school girls, lived in the same dormitory room, and helped each other study for a long time now. What they shared was truly sisterly love for each other. And Misti needed all the family she had.

Three

By the end of Misti's second week in the Shock Trauma Unit, the nurses had begun doing some basic physical therapy with her. At first they just rubbed her legs and arms to stimulate the circulation and then moved her fingers and hands, and elbows, knees, and ankles to maintain muscle tone and keep the joints from locking. The hospital's physical therapy department had made plaster casts for her feet and legs. The casts were sawed in half length-wise; the pieces were then put on Misti's legs and secured with elastic bandages on a schedule of two hours on, two hours off to try to counteract the shortening of her tendons and the twisting of her limbs. Misti, still deep in her coma, did not appear to notice and certainly did not object.

The nurses at the STU had begun to regard Misti's boyfriend, Max, as a member of the immediate family; they knew he would not do or say anything to upset Misti. He came to visit her as often as he could— just about every day immediately after school. Fortunately, his school was nearby, and since he was a day scholar, rather than a boarding student, he did not have to worry about getting off-campus leave. He was very gentle with Misti, and he always talked to her about his dog, who Misti loved, and how he was doing in school, and about their mutual friends. One day, as Max and I were standing on opposite sides of Misti's bed and talking, I noticed that her head seemed to be moving slightly, turning from one of us to the other as we spoke. Her eyes were still closed, but it seemed to me that she was following our voices. I did not mention this to Max, though, for fear of getting his hopes up. As we left Misti's room, I let Max go on ahead, then stopped at the nurses' station and told the nurse on duty what I thought I'd just witnessed. A moment later, she was heading into Misti's room to check for herself. I also let Harry know about Misti's movements that evening, and then we both tried not to hope too much that things might be starting to improve for Misti. At the same time, I was absolutely convinced that she was going to recover. Since God had not seen fit to take her right after the accident, he clearly had another plan for her, and that surely would involve recovery.

Meanwhile, every time she seemed to be making some progress toward stability, there would be some sort of setback. For instance, Misti kept spiking fevers—from no clear source, but probably the result of an infection in one of the IV lines or catheters—and she was started on antibiotics. She was still on a respirator at this point and was fed via glucose IVs.

As part of the daily STU routine, the nurses and doctors kept checking Misti's reflexes and asking her to open her eyes, squeeze their hands, move her foot—just to see whether she was capable of making some kind of reflex response on command. The responses were very intermittent; one day she would be able to respond weakly when asked to raise a finger, the next day she lay there totally still. The doctors were careful to caution us that any response was purely reflex.

Her eyes were sometimes half-open, but again the doctors said this was no indication that she was actually returning to consciousness. The nurses asked me which television programs she liked to watch, and when I told them that Misti was a real soap opera fan, they wheeled a TV into Misti's room so that *The Young and the Restless* and *General Hospital* could be tuned in. The theory behind this kind of stimulation, they said, is that the injured and recovering brain is more likely to respond to familiar sounds, sights, and even smells than to new ones.

At the suggestion of Mr. Jones, the chaplain at Mercersburg, Misti's classmates had recorded audiotapes to be played for her. It was terribly touching to listen to their young voices trying to be upbeat and cheerful, telling Misti about the latest gossip and what was happening in various classes and on the school's athletic teams. We later learned that Mr. Jones had made the kids practice and retape their messages so that Misti wouldn't hear any fear or sadness in their voices. Each day we read to Misti from the dozens of cards and letters she was receiving and told her who was visiting in the waiting room and who had called. Harry and I were careful to keep Misti up to date on the activities of her brothers and her nieces and nephew, and we filled the cork board message center in her room with pictures of family and friends. We talked to her about everything and anything. One day, I remember, I told Misti that I hoped she wouldn't choose that particular day to come out of her coma because she'd see that I was wearing a sweater she'd always hated.

In less than a month, life had changed drastically. Gone were the demands of home and work, the pleasures of reading, pursuing hobbies, or just spending time with family and friends. Now life was waking up in the morning grateful that Misti was still breathing and hopeful that today she would regain consciousness. We were at the hospital until 8:00 P.M. every day. Then we'd head "home" to the hotel to make the first call in the phone chain and report on the day's events. We made sure that the nurses had our number and asked that they call us with any change, any news, good or bad.

Despite our exhaustion and the comfort of our hotel, night never brought much rest for either Harry or me. I had recurrent nightmares in which I was trying to hold back the tractor trailer that was about to hit Misti. Harry was also very restless—usually up half of the night, pacing up and down. Any phone call at night brought terror, but one particular midnight, the voice at the other end of the line finally brought some encouragement. The call was from a nurse in the STU, who told us that she was certain that Misti had squeezed her hand slightly in response to her request and seemed to be responding to Odette's voice on the tapes. Very excited that something positive was finally starting to happen, we called Chuck and Cork with the news. After that night, I never told myself that I shouldn't be too hopeful. There were plenty of people at the hospital who were in the business of being cautious. My feeling was that God had promised that Misti would get better—and this gave me the confidence I needed to keep going.

The next day as I stood by her bedside, Misti moved her right hand as if in protest when one of the doctors lifted her eyelid. Her right leg also started a series of jerks, quick and involuntary. I was thrilled, but the doctor said these were reflexes that would take place even though Misti was in deep coma; it was the responses she made to requests that were important.

Misti's medical condition continued to wax and wane from day to day. One day, she seemed to be responsive, the next, too exhausted to make any effort at all. For the most part, her eyes were shut. In some respects, the doctors seemed to have less hope as time went on, probably because the coma was so profound. Further, Misti was still spiking the occasional fever and had a bad case of digestive upset. Her blood work was showing that she was still diabetic, a sign that her injured brain was not yet allowing her metabolism to work properly.

Then, little by little, Misti's physical condition seemed to stabilize and then improve. Although she was still in a world of her own, the doctors now agreed that she was getting closer to holding her own. By the end of Misti's third week in the STU, they decided that it was time to remove the brain probe. They explained that it was still impossible to know the extent of brain damage. Eventually, after all the swelling had gone down and the blood clots resolved, a magnetic resonance imaging (MRI) test would show how much of the brain had been damaged and where the damage was. When the bandage was removed from the top of Misti's head, we were amazed to see a crop of thick new hair growing on her scalp.

Once they were convinced her condition had truly stabilized, the doctors began to talk about getting Misti ready to leave the STU, which meant weaning her from the respirator and placing a tube to her stomach through her nose so that she could be fed without intravenous lines. And since Misti was no longer in immediate danger, we would need to find a new facility for her; she could not be kept in the STU once she no longer needed acute care. Nor would it do much good to release her into the main hospital, they said, because on a regular ward, Misti would not get the constant therapy she would need if she was to have any chance at recovery. It really would be best, the social services staff told us, for Misti to be put in a head trauma facility for rehabilitation, if one would take her. The other option was a "long-term care facility," which, I learned, was a sugar-coated way of saying a nursing home.

Harry and I felt that we'd been given no real choice. We would not consider placing Misti in a nursing home, where she would have gotten custodial care at best, rather than the active therapy that would be necessary to help her regain her functions. Having watched some of Misti's care in the STU and having helped my mother with the care of my father, I knew that I wasn't equipped to take care of Misti at home. So, since the hospital staff insisted that plans must be made for Misti to leave, Harry and I set out to find out about head trauma rehabilitation hospitals in the area. The staff at Suburban said they would help us in any way they could, and fortunately, between our own insurance and the state of Pennsylvania's catastrophic accident fund (CAT fund), which covered all of the state's licensed drivers, we would be able to afford good care for her.

With the help of one of the hospital's social workers, Harry and I put together a list of possibilities in Pennsylvania, hoping to find an appropriate facility near our home in Waynesboro. Harry and the social worker made appointments for us, then we gathered maps and planned a blitzkrieg day trip to look at the three most likely places. The first stop was the rehab ward at Mechanicsburg Hospital. The hospital had the advantage of being less than forty miles away from Waynesboro, but the facility seemed to be set up for mostly for elderly stroke victims. We saw only a few young people with brain injury there, and they were tied into their wheelchairs, with their unsupported heads drooping forward and spittle falling from their open mouths. This was the first time that I had seen people with traumatic brain injury outside of the STU, and the realization that this might be Misti's fate was brutal. Until that point, I had not really allowed myself to think about what the limits of "rehabilitation" might be. I could not imagine Misti there.

From Mechanicsburg, we went on to a facility in Reading, which was even further from home. Though the initial shock had begun to wear off, I had a bad reaction to this place, too. It was an old, red brick building that looked like a castle; because of a renovation project, the corridors and lobby were draped in plastic and full of plaster dust, with workmen going about their jobs. And though it was being modernized, the building still retained the worst of hospital smells—that unmistakable mix of disinfectant and stale urine. The halls were crowded and noisy, with mostly older people propped up in wheelchairs screaming or groaning. The entire place felt shabby and depressing, conveying an air of hopelessness. It was certainly not a place that inspired hope in the possibility of rehabilitation, certainly not a place for Misti.

As Harry and I traveled through the Pennsylvania countryside, heading toward the last of the rehab facilities on our list, we discussed what we would do if we didn't find anything suitable in the area. We had hoped Misti could be cared for near home, but we were willing to take her out of state if that proved necessary. We had been hearing about a wonderful facility in California, and that became our escape hatch. We were determined that Misti should have the best chance possible at full recovery, and if that meant moving with her to California and forgoing visits from friends and family, then that was what we would do.

The last place on our list—Bryn Mawr Rehabilitation Hospital, located not in Bryn Mawr but on the Paoli Pike in Malvern—was about four hours from home, too far for many of Misti's friends to be able to visit easily when she was able to have visitors. Along the way, I was startled to see a sign for Goshen Road, and without conscious thought, my mind flew back to the accident that had taken place on Midcounty Highway and Goshen Road a month before. So much had changed since then.

We drove down the road a short distance and turned right. Before us was a modern hospital building set on very well-kept grounds with lots of trees and a fountain. A great flock of Canadian geese were on the grounds, probably attracted by the large pond out in the back. As we drove down the long access road, I began to feel hope rising again. Maybe this was the right place for Misti. At the Rehab, Harry and I were met by extremely polite, smiling people. Unlike the other places we had seen, which seemed gloomy and forbidding, this place was light and bright, and Harry and I immediately felt comfortable. The staff members were clearly friendly, and amazingly, everyone seemed to smile. As we walked through the facility, we noticed that on the doors to each room were the patients' names, each with the title of Mr., Mrs., or Miss. How great, I said, the patients here are treated with dignity. I was politely corrected by our guide: "Here we refer to them as guests." Taking in the bright, cheerful hallways, the clean rooms with their views of the rolling countryside, the busy and impressive therapy areas, I felt confident that this place would bring Misti back to us.

Harry and I met with the administrators, discussing Misti's condition and our hopes and expectations—and of course, the matter of our insurance and what it would cover. It was agreed that Bryn Mawr's doctors would speak to Misti's doctors in Bethesda, then review their findings with the Bryn Mawr board. But if we got the approval of the rehab specialists from Bryn Mawr and the okay from the insurance people, we could have Misti transferred shortly.

As we left, we saw a young man in a wheelchair with his arms hanging down uselessly, pushing himself with his feet. I found myself praying, "Please God, let Misti be able to do that someday." All her past life and abilities were now forgotten; life now existed in a new form. It's remarkable how quickly life can change. Only a few weeks ago I had been sure that Misti would change the world as a doctor. Now my hope was that someday she could learn to propel her own wheelchair. When the worst thing that can happen already has, the simplest things become wonderful.

Max's parents had offered to stay with Misti while Harry and I looked at rehab facilities, and they had let Max take the day off from school to visit with her so she wouldn't get panicky at the change in routine. They were anxious to hear what we'd found. But first they told us that Richard Winslow had been charged with failing to yield the right of way and been fined forty dollars. For the first time since the accident, I gave in to my emotions. "Can you even fathom that a man does this to our lovely daughter, changes the lives of everyone in our family so completely, destroys so many dreams, and he pays a fine of forty dollars? Why bother? The man certainly can't have much of a conscience. He has never even so much as called to see how she is. He never walked into the hospital to inquire if she even survived his carelessness." I am not usually one to question why things happen, but that day I did. "For heaven's sake, forty dollars for altering so many lives. Forty dollars will not even make him think twice. He just goes on his merry way, doing his job, his life not at all disrupted, with no apparent sense of guilt." Harry and Brenda and Anthony could only voice their agreement. Not only was the sentence out of proportion to the act, but it would certainly prove no deterrent to anyone or prod any careless driver into greater vigilance.

Once I calmed down, Harry and I told Brenda and Anthony what the administrators at Bryn Mawr Rehabilitation had said: In order to be admitted to Bryn Mawr, a patient must be responding to treatment and have left the critical care unit. If there was a chance that the patient would need any kind of acute care, he or she would not be accepted by Bryn Mawr, which was not a hospital, but a rehabilitation center. This meant that the schedule to get Misti weaned from the respirator and moved from IV onto nasogastric feeding would have to be accelerated. Harry and I were sure that if we could just get Bryn Mawr to accept Misti, she would recover and come back to us. It might take a while, but certainly it would happen.

Now the pace at the STU picked up dramatically. Perhaps sensing a change in my attitude, perhaps trying to prepare me for the next phase of our lives, the nurses asked whether I was interested in learning to help with Misti's various therapies. My instincts to help had been thwarted for weeks, as I had to stand back and let professionals take over, and I immediately felt better once this arrangement was in place. There was another incentive in this: If I learned Misti's therapy, I could stay with her much of the day and be of real help. I was thrilled at the prospect. No longer would I have to wait for the always too-short visits. Harry, needing the same sense that he too was doing something concrete, decided to return to Waynesboro and help Chuck and Cork as he had promised when the sale of the businesses went through. Harry has always been an active man, a doer, and the waiting was taking a heavy toll on him. And, of course, there was the problem of money. Bryn Mawr was certainly a wonderful facility, and even with good insurance and the help of the state's CAT fund, Misti's care there was going to cost money. Part of the plan behind selling the Morningstar businesses to Chuck and Cork had always been for Harry to get started in real estate development, and now he would. This would involve a lot of hard work, but if it were successful, it would certainly help take care of Misti's needs.

Once I became involved with her care, I began to see that at times Misti moved her right arm quite a bit. Eventually, it became necessary to use restraints to keep her from pulling out the various tubes and IV lines. One day when I left to take a short break, she worked her hand free and pulled out her breathing tube, setting off alarms that brought the nurses running. The doctor in the unit at the time put an oxygen mask over Misti's mouth and nose and waited, hoping to avoid having to cut into her airway and insert a tracheotomy tube. "I really don't want to cut a trache in this girl's neck," he said. "She's so beautiful, and I don't want her to have another scar." I took his statement as a sign of his belief that she was going to recover enough to care about having visible reminders of this experience, and fortunately, the tracheotomy proved unnecessary.

The following day Misti lay very still; clearly, the previous day's excitement with the tube had exhausted her. The nurses tried in vain to get her to move her head or her arm or hand. This was one of the days when she seemed to step back, rather than moving toward recovery. Though they were almost ready to discharge her, the doctors still would not even venture a guess at her chances of full recovery. After her previous advances, the situation that day was very discouraging. I wondered what the burn-out rate of nurses in this unit must be. Each seemed to care so much and to work so diligently for each patient, and when I stopped to think just how few of these patients would ever recover and how limited that recovery might be, the nurses' diligence and compassion seemed nothing short of miraculous.

As I talked to Misti that afternoon, rubbing her pale, thin arms and legs, I begged her to open her eyes. But not the twitch of a muscle or even a sigh told me that she had heard me. I wondered how long she might continue to lie in a coma with no sign of recovery, no promises, almost no hope.

That night I came across an Ann Landers column with the headline, "A poem for parents coping with loss of a child." The popular columnist was sharing a poem with a mother who had recently lost her twenty-four-month-old son. The poem had been written by Edgar A. Guest, and once I started reading, I could not keep from going on.

"For All Parents"

I'll lend you for a little time, a child of mine, he said.
For you to love while he lives and mourn when he is dead.
It may be six or seven years or twenty-two or three.
But will you, till I call him back, take care of him for me?
He'll bring his charm to gladden you, and shall his stay be brief,
You'll have his lovely memories as solace for your grief.
I cannot promise he will stay, since all from earth return.
But there are lessons taught down there I want this child to learn.
I've looked the wide world over in my search for teachers true,
And from the throngs that crowd life's lanes, I have selected you.
Now will you give him all your love, nor think the labor vain,
Nor hate me when I come to call to take him back again?
I fancied that I heard them say, Dear Lord, thy will be done.
For all the joy thy child shall bring, the risk of grief we'll run.

We'll shelter him with tenderness, we'll love him while we may,
And for the happiness we've known, will ever grateful stay.
But shall the angels call for him much sooner than we planned,
We'll brave the bitter grief that comes and try to understand.

I found myself near tears. If Misti had died, we would have been devastated with grief and mourned deeply. But Misti was not dead, yet she was not quite alive, either. I was mourning not her death, but a life that could have been. I would not give up now, however. I was resolved that however dark things looked at present, Misti would recover.

The STU nurses and social workers did their best to bring my hopes down, to make me think more realistically. They were certain that the sooner I accepted the fact that it was not possible for Misti to recover in any real way, the sooner I would be able to make realistic plans for Misti and the rest of the family and get on with life. Once again, they explained that Misti's brain had been badly bruised and torn up on initial impact, and then, as the seat belt restrained Misti's body, her head continued forward, causing the brain to bounce forward to the front of the skull (in brain-injury parlance, this first blow is known as the "coup"). Then when her head hit the windshield and the seat broke loose, the whiplash forced her head back, and the brain bounced back toward the rear of the skull (the "countrecoup"). My head started to spin under the relentless assault of this medical explanation. The bottom line was that Misti's brain had been so severely damaged that medically, recovery was impossible. Even if she continued to breathe and her heart continued to beat—which would happen as long as her brain stem was intact—she would only exist in "a persistent vegetative state."

Clearly, they thought rehabilitation was an impossibility, that Misti would remain in a coma forever. What if that were the case? Would she want to live like this? Was there any quality to the life she was living now? Should we pull the plugs and donate Misti's organs? If she never recovered to any greater extent, where would the money come from to keep her alive? And the final question, would the money we were planning to spend on rehabilitation be better spent on research for brain trauma treatment?

Uncontrollable tears flooded my eyes later that evening as I asked Harry whether he realized what the world lost when Misti's brain was injured. Even rationalizing that a young girl's dreams do not always come true, the world would certainly lose a great deal if she did not recover. With all the courage and love and confidence he could summon, Harry took me in his arms and assured me that Misti would recover.

Max was still visiting as often as the hospital would allow. Each time he entered Misti's room, he clasped the gold bracelet he had bought her for Valentine's Day about her thin wrist. Since hospital policy dictated that no valuables be left with the patient, the nurses made him remove it and take it away with him each time he left. Max had also brought Misti a white stuffed bear, whose tag read "Party Bear," to keep Misti company when he could not be there. One day, Max picked up the diary we'd been using for progress notes and wrote, "Happy eight-month anniversary, Misti. Love, Max." His love, dedication, and devotion were touching in one so young; no one could have anticipated that he would be spending the spring of his junior year of high school shuttling between his classes and Misti's bedside.

Dr. Jamshidi, who had performed the original surgery on Misti's brain, decided it was time for a follow-up EEG to measure her brain waves and the efficacy of the antiseizure medicine. When the results came in, both he and the STU internist reported themselves happy with Misti's progress. The medicine she was being given was keeping the seizures under control, and the EEG showed that there was some return of well-organized brain activity. A few days later, one of the nurses from the STU came running into the waiting room where Harry and I were sitting. She seemed terribly excited and asked us to follow her quickly. As we neared Misti's glass-walled room, we could see what she was so excited about: Through the glass walls we could see Misti moving her left hand a little. The nurse told us that when she had changed the bed and replaced the diaper she now wore, Misti had seemed to lift her body to help with the change. The nurse then lifted Misti out of bed and put her into a bedside chair, with the stuffed bear beside her. For the first time, Misti seemed to be trying to keep her eyes open for more than a few seconds at a time.

Hope flared anew. Misti had been nearly unresponsive only days before, but now she was sitting in a chair. When one of the occupational therapists made her rounds later that day, she noted in the diary: "Misti was sitting in the chair today, head leaning to the right, unable to maintain her head upright. Eyes opened slightly for brief periods. Held on to 'Party Bear' while eyes opened. Squeezed right hand upon command. Appears pretty tired today." But this terse, deliberately low-key report represented real progress, and we all knew it.

Now as the occupational therapists worked with Misti, they described everything they were doing, giving directions: Up, down, touch your nose, cheek, etc. Even though Misti was not always responsive, everyone made an effort to treat her as though she were able to hear everything. I witnessed further progress a few days afterward, when Misti held onto a small round plastic tube, giving slight resistance when we tried to remove it from her hand.

A month after the accident, Misti's condition had improved significantly. She had been weaned from the ventilator, she was no longer running fevers, she seemed to follow voices and could occasionally comply with simple commands, and she was able to sit up in a chair—albeit with anchoring restraints—to receive visitors. Although the nurses told us that much of what we were seeing was pure reflex action, we were elated. Call it what they might, Misti was making progress. There would be no stopping her now.

Four

It took Bryn Mawr a week or so to confirm that they would accept Misti. As soon as we got word of their decision, Harry and I started working with the nurses to have Misti transferred to a regular ward at Suburban to demonstrate that she no longer needed the special services of the Shock Trauma Unit. This was essential, since Bryn Mawr's policy was not to admit patients directly from critical care.

Later that week, Harry and I took a very early morning trip to Bryn Mawr to make the necessary arrangements to move Misti. We learned that she would be placed on Unit 700, where all coma patients with traumatic brain injury started out, and we agreed that Misti would have the benefits of a Bryn Mawr bed—a special bed fashioned from an open-topped, fully padded wooden box. The Bryn Mawr bed came with a king-sized mattress at the bottom and walls about four feet high. The front wall had a hinged gate that opened out for access and could be closed to provide safety. This ingenious bed had been developed for brain trauma patients at Bryn Mawr and allowed family members and caretakers to maintain close body contact with and provide stimulation to the patient recovering from coma. In her Bryn Mawr bed, Misti would not have to be restrained when she started to come out of the coma. Instead, she would be able to move freely—even thrash around—without hurting herself, and thus might be able to recover more quickly.

With years of experience in dealing with traumatic brain injury patients and their families, the Bryn Mawr personnel were all very gentle as they explained to us that if—and they put strong emphasis on the conditional—Misti were to come out of the coma, she would pass through many stages as she recovered. I found myself blocking out most of what the rehab specialists were trying so hard to tell me because it all sounded so horrible. I was still clinging desperately to my Hollywood image of recovery from coma. Maybe, I thought to myself, Misti would prove the exception to what I was beginning to recognize as the rule. I was also beginning to realize that recovery from coma for Misti might mean that the girl who had once dreamed of being a professional dancer might be confined to a wheelchair.

The week before Misti's transfer to Bryn Mawr, her roommate Odette was given permission by the Academy to spend the weekend with us. We were expecting that Misti would be moved up to Bryn Mawr any time now, and we knew that once the move had taken place, Odette would have a much harder time traveling to see Misti.

Odette spent the time with Misti almost the same way she would have in the dorm room at Mercersburg. She chattered away to Misti the entire time about typical girl stuff—what was going on in their classes and who was going out with whom. She also used the time she was allowed to put twenty-five braids in Misti's hair. One of the nurses told us that although Misti was not terribly responsive to what Odette was saying, she did seem to be moving her head slightly as if to look around to see the source of the sound.

In the meantime, plans to move Misti were becoming more concrete. An ambulance with an attendant and all the necessary medical equipment would carry her to Bryn Mawr. The trip would take between three and a half and four hours. The nurses and doctors at Suburban thought that I should ride along with her. They were not sure whether or not Misti was aware of her surroundings, but if she were, she might find the ambulance ride very confusing. Since she seemed responsive to sound, they thought it might comfort her if she could hear my voice.

At 8:00 A.M. on the day of Misti's move, a very cheerful young man came into Misti's new room with an ambulance stretcher. With the help of one of the nurses, we transferred Misti from her bed to his stretcher, then made sure we had all her personal items, such as the photographs and cards we'd been collecting and the stuffed bear that Max had given her. The nurse reminded me that I had to go to the hospital's office to sign the final papers for Misti's release, then gave me a hug. With her "Good luck" ringing in my ears, I left for the office.

I have never had a stranger experience than going into the office, signing Misti's release papers, and being told to pick up her personal effects in the back room. There, I was handed a plastic bag containing two gold necklaces, several gold rings, and a wristwatch. Quite unexpectedly, memories flooded over me; it was as if I was looking at Misti's past, a life she might never know again. Distantly, I heard someone say something about these few things being all that was left because Misti's clothing had all been cut away. This was all that was left—this and the injury that had robbed her of the life she had known.

☺

The back of the ambulance was small and crowded. With Misti positioned on the driver's side with her head facing the front of the ambulance, there was not much room along the opposite side for the attendant and me to sit comfortably. The attendant got to his knees in the cramped space and looked up into my face, observing, "You don't smile very much."

"Well, really, it's not as though I have a lot to smile about," I said, and then realized that my reply had been just short of rude.

Undaunted, he promised, "Before we get to Philadelphia you will smile." He then proceeded to sing, offering his impressions, first of Dean Martin and then Frank Sinatra. His impersonations were extremely good, and before long he had me not only smiling, but laughing. By the time he started to do Elvis, even Misti had a hint of a smile. Because of the brain damage, only one side of her mouth—the right side—moved, but half a smile was just fine with me. This was the first time she had displayed any emotion since the accident, and I was convinced that it showed real progress.

The funny thing was that Misti had always disliked Elvis and refused to listen to his records. Here in the ambulance, she was a captive audience. She must be able to hear, I decided. Why else would she smile at the attendant's soulful rendition of "Love Me Tender"? Thinking that this might be one of her lucid moments, I seized the opportunity to explain to Misti that we were leaving the hospital because she was doing so well, that Bryn Mawr was the place where she would recover, that she would soon be talking and walking and going back to school. Then I kissed her cheek and told her that I loved her. The attendant put his hand on mine and said, "If anything ever happens to me, I hope you can be there to help. This girl is going to make it. I feel the vibes. Man, do I feel the vibes." I fervently hoped that he was right.

In what seemed to be no time at all, we arrived at Bryn Mawr, where the staff was waiting to welcome Misti. She was quickly moved out of the ambulance and installed in her room in Unit 700. The ward held nine or ten glass-fronted rooms arranged around a central nurses' station. Misti's room was bright and cheerful. The large picture window here offered a view of a small lake with a fountain and made the place feel more like a pleasant home than a hospital. The nursing staff made Misti comfortable in her Bryn Mawr bed, and for the first time since the accident, she seemed truly peaceful. Soon she was sleeping, with Max lying beside her in the fenced-in bed, holding her hand.

Leaving Misti under Max's watchful eye, Harry and I took a more detailed tour of the rehab facility, which included a nice cafeteria for staff and family members, a top-notch gym for physical therapy, a small chapel, and a gift shop. Then we returned to the brain trauma unit and became acquainted with the nurses there. Peggy would be Misti's primary daytime nurse, taking major care of her. Linda would keep on top of all of the scheduling—the therapies and evaluations, the meals, and the events in the rehab. The very quiet and extremely patient Betty would be the third member of the day team. Other nurses would take care of Misti at night, and, of course, there would be new people rotating through on weekends and during vacations.

The next day, we filled out more of the endless papers necessary and met the therapists who would be working with Misti—Karen, the physical therapist; Terry, the occupational therapist; Cyndy, the speech pathologist; and Maria Scotto, the clinical psychologist who would be monitoring Misti's progress in cognitive retraining once we got to that stage.

That afternoon, there was a planning conference for us, so that we would know what Misti's rehabilitation would involve. We met the social workers who would be working with us, Dr. Audieh, the head of the medical team, and a variety of other support people. Barbara Wesson, the director of Bryn Mawr, asked me what we wanted to happen in the next few months. Well, I said, that was simple. We wanted them to bring Misti back to us fully restored, and then for her to return to Mercersburg and graduate from the Academy, then go on to college and live a wonderful life, happy forever after. Oh, and they should please bring her back from the coma as a neat person; she had always been a bit messy, and since they'd asked what I'd like, I would like that to change. As I finished, I studied the stunned looks on the faces of the rehab specialists. I watched them turn to Harry, hoping for a more sensible response. I realized that they had not picked up on my joke, my reaction to being asked, after the previous long and dreadful month, what I actually might want.

Clearly, there would have to be some adjustments made. Although the staff at Bryn Mawr had dealt with many families with high hopes, they did not yet know me or Harry. We'd spent the last month walking a tightrope between hope and dread, and the bottom line was that we wanted everything possible done for our daughter, no matter how hopeless the situation might look at present. The meeting ended soon after that, with members of the staff sort of nodding at us as we left.

⑨

Without much formal discussion, Harry and I had agreed that the only sensible plan was for me to stay with Misti while he went back to Waynesboro to help Chuck and Cork and to start working on the new ventures that he had planned. He would be able to stay for a few days now and would try to get back up here as often as possible. Neither of us was happy at the prospect of so much separation, but the issue was Misti's survival and recovery, not what we might have preferred.

The staff at our hotel in Bethesda had made arrangements for us at a sister facility in nearby Valley Forge, and we hoped that that would be our base while Misti was at Bryn Mawr Rehab, but our room there proved much smaller than our room in Bethesda had been. We didn't know how long we would be here, but if we were going to need a home away from home for an extended period of time, it had to be more comfortable and welcoming. Perhaps, we thought, we could locate a furnished house or apartment, with everything necessary to be comfortable for a few months.

Luck was with us. A few hours later, a woman behind the counter in a local real estate office mentioned that a furnished townhouse in a nearby development that was owned by a supermarket chain and kept available for their traveling executives. The property was now on the market for sale, but the supermarket people had not mentioned the possibility of renting it. Grasping at any chance—I had to get this settled so I could get back to Misti—I found myself asking her to call and find out not whether they would rent it, but for how much. The realtor's inquiry revealed that the supermarket chain would indeed be willing to rent the Chesterbrook townhouse to me until it was sold. This meant that the realtor's lock would always be on the front door and that I would have to make sure the place was in shape to be shown at any time; and of course, once it was sold, I would have to move immediately. I said this sounded fair to me.

I moved in the next day. The townhouse was a tastefully decorated three-level model with a wonderful kitchen, a dining room with lots of mirrors, a fireplace, and patio doors that opened onto a deck. In addition to a master bedroom and bath there was a guest room and a den with a TV. It would make a wonderful place to come home to at the end of each day. And with the guest room and den, there would be plenty of space if the boys or their families—or Max, or any other friends, for that matter—wanted to come up over the weekend and visit Misti.

At the end of the weekend, Harry finally had to leave to return to Waynesboro. Chuck had driven the family's second car, a small Pontiac, up to Malvern for me, and he would go back with Harry. It was very hard for Harry to leave Misti largely in the hands of strangers, no matter how well-trained and pleasant, and it was hard for both of us to part. In the past month, we'd been each other's strongest support, one offering encouragement when the other was down, and though the move to Bryn Mawr represented progress for Misti, the separation was going to be hard on the two of us. But we each had our tasks. Our goal was to help Misti get better, and we would do whatever was necessary to that end.

⊚

Misti's early days at Bryn Mawr were taken up with evaluation by the various doctors and therapists. I worried about the conclusions they would draw because it took days for Misti to recover from the stress of the transfer. As we had learned, the recovering brain requires a great deal of rest. In addition, Misti was still taking Dilantin, a strong anti-seizure medication, which added to her drowsiness. It was discouraging to note that after the strides she'd made during the last week at Suburban, she seemed to be showing almost no response to the therapists or to me. Perhaps, I reflected, we should not have been so hasty in making the move to Bryn Mawr, but what was done could not be undone, and we now had to make the best of the situation.

The first order of business was to learn the ward's routine. Unlike in the hospital, where the nurses had kept her draped, but not really dressed, in open-backed hospital gowns, Misti was now to be dressed in sweat suits, which were easy to put on and remove and would keep her warm and covered as she became more active. Each day, there would be therapy sessions in the mornings and afternoons, with time out for lunch. Since Misti was still being fed via a nasogastric tube, she was excused from meals in the patients' dining room for the present. For now, therapy—range of motion exercises, sitting up in a chair, the first steps toward speech and swallowing therapy—would take place in Misti's room, but she would soon be going to regular sessions in the gym and other therapy rooms. Eventually there would be water therapy and even therapy involving horseback riding. (Misti would be riding horses? I wondered, looking down at her still form. Maybe this would indeed be a place of miracles.) In the evenings, various recreational activities, such as movies and "pet therapy," were offered. (Pet therapy was a particularly innovative technique that had gotten some surprisingly good results. The process involved introducing the patient to cats, dogs, rabbits and other small animals to stimulate their recovery. Unfortunately, due to animal allergies, Misti was not able to take advantage of this therapy.) As to personal grooming, Peggy explained that Misti would be given a shower three times a week—Monday, Wednesday, and Friday; the every-other-day schedule was necessary because of the number of patients and the time it took to shower each.

As we prepared Misti for her first shower, the nurse brought in a rubber stretcher with holes punched in the sling section. The procedure involved transferring Misti to the stretcher, covering her with a large towel, then wheeling her into the shower room, a tiled room approximately eleven feet by eleven feet. The concrete floor slanted down toward a central drain, and a hose with a shower head hung from the ceiling. The whole set-up reminded me of a car wash. The nurse adjusted the shower head, and then, for the first time in a month, Misti had a shower, the warm soapy water running off into the drain. In the process, all three of us got soaked; I could certainly see why a somewhat restricted showering schedule was necessary. Not surprisingly, Misti seemed to enjoy the shower very much; after all, this was the girl who would often take two showers and wash her hair every day. This must feel quite different from the sponge baths at Suburban. As we watched her sleep after the shower, it seemed to me that she was resting much more easily, her restless right arm very still and a look of contentment on her face.

☺

Early the next morning, the drive to the Rehab took me through a beautiful landscape. A soft snow had fallen and glistened like silver. After greeting Misti, who seemed to be asleep, I lay down beside her in the Bryn Mawr bed. Then suddenly, she opened her eyes, looked at me, and said matter-of-factly, "I think we should go home now." A rush of joy flooded my mind; then I was catapulted out of this rosy dream into wakefulness. Struggling to awareness, I heard the patients' cries and institutional noises. Misti's voice had been echoing in my mind, but now it slipped away, leaving me to look at her drawn face, her motionless body, her twisted arms and legs. It's one thing to mourn death, but for the last month, I had been mourning life, a life that could have been. Numbly, I closed my eyes and started praying, "Our Father, who art in heaven. . . ." At the end of the prayer, I found myself repeating, "Thy will be done, Thy will be done . . . ." Then I swore at God.

Moments later, I looked up as Linda walked into the room. Although Bryn Mawr is a nonsectarian facility, the practice was to write a bible verse on the scheduling boards in patients' rooms each day. It's been said that as long as there are fourth graders with math tests, there will always be prayers in schools, and the same rules apply to hospitals and rehab facilities. Now Linda scrawled the message for today: "With God all things are possible." Seeing my tear-stained face, Linda sat down beside me, offering the thought that the accident was not God's doing, that sometimes even God cannot stop the adversary, but that God does have a role in recovery. As we talked, I began to realize that God must have known this accident was going to happen and in many ways had prepared the way for us to help Misti recover from it. For instance, we had recently traded in an attractive but unreliable Cadillac for a sturdier Lincoln. On the way home from the dealer, we had laughed about our impulsive buy. I realized now that if we still owned the Cadillac the long trips that Harry would be making from Waynesboro to Bryn Mawr each weekend would be impossible. Similarly, if something bad had to happen to Misti, this was probably the best time for it. Our lives were in very good shape. Cork and Chuck were independent and doing well, the businesses had been transferred, Harry and I were in good health. We hadn't known when we were making plans for this period of our lives that we'd need the decks cleared to take good care of Misti, but that was how things had worked out. After my bout of anger at God, the verse on the board and my conversation with Linda offered reassurance that even though I doubt sometimes, God would always be there, taking care of us.

The next day, I woke to the conviction that this day would be better than the previous. As the saying goes, this was the first day of the rest of my life. I drove out of Chesterbrook and headed for the highway, thinking optimistically about what I had accomplished lately. Here I was, a person who never drove on highways, nonchalantly driving to the Paoli Pike for another day in the Rehab.

As I entered Misti's room, I was pleasantly surprised to see her hand extended above the top of the Bryn Mawr bed. I quickly opened the gate and crawled in with her. She was holding her right arm almost straight up, and her right leg was moving. Although she did not seem to be looking at anything in particular—in fact, one eye was looking straight ahead while the other was looking off at an angle—both eyes were definitely open. Perhaps she had begun to recover from the ambulance ride at last.

Immediately, I lay down beside Misti and started talking to her. The nurses and the booklets on traumatic brain injury had explained that talking to her and touching her were the best things we could do to help her emerge from the coma. For the next several hours, I talked to her about the Academy, her friends, our neighbors, past vacations, pets we had had, and family events, stroking her arms all the while. Although she seemed to be responding somewhat, we still did not know for sure how much damage her brain had sustained, so there was no way of knowing how much was getting through.

Later that morning, Karen, the physical therapist, arrived to take measurements for adapting a wheelchair especially for Misti. Even though I had heard at one of the meetings that this would be done quickly, I was still surprised when Misti's customized wheelchair was brought in the very next day. I was a little bit afraid that Misti wasn't really ready for a wheelchair, that it might be dangerous for her because she had so little control over her body, but this chair had a rod up the back and a halo structure on top to hold her head. A band of Velcro straps attached the halo to her head. The chair came with a clear acrylic tray strapped to its arms so that Misti's arms and hands could rest comfortably. A rubber restraint that reminded me of a rolling pin would go across her lap to hold her body in an erect position. Like the Bryn Mawr bed, the customized wheelchair confirmed for me that the staff at Bryn Mawr were indeed professionals who knew their jobs very well. And I was happy to see that once Misti was in the chair, with its protective apparatus, her head was held erect, unlike the brain injured patients we'd seen at the other rehabilitative facilities. This not only made her look much more normal, but it gave us greater hope that recovery was possible.

Once Misti's new wheelchair was available, we were able to get her out of her room, both for therapies and for the stimulation of a change of scene. First, however, we weighed her. She was down to only 117 pounds from her pre-accident weight of 135 pounds. Clearly, we had to build her back up. Next, we went to the X-ray room. Dr. Audieh had observed that in addition to suffering foot drop, Misti seemed to be holding her left ankle at a somewhat odd angle, and she wanted to make sure that there was not a fracture that had been overlooked. When this proved not to be the case, we got the okay to start therapy, though we were told that Misti might need a new cast for that ankle.

When a new therapist, Cathy, came into the room to perform a swallowing evaluation, I was worried, not sure how she could make any real judgments because Misti seemed to be asleep throughout the entire test. But Cathy knew her job, and told me that in order for swallow therapy (the precursor to both eating and speech therapy) to begin, Misti must be sitting up in the chair. So the goal for the moment was to see that Misti would spend more time in the chair on each successive day. This often meant fighting Misti's clear desire to go back to bed and sleep, but it was essential for recovery. It was fascinating to learn that while some forms of therapy would have to wait until Misti was further out of the coma, other forms of therapy, such as sitting, massage, and stimulation of the senses, could begin immediately.

Even though the physical therapists had started to do range of motion therapy with Misti, they were still putting the casts on her arms and legs. Now, however, the casts remained on all night as well as at intervals throughout the day. Within short order, the physical therapy team had decided that Misti needed a new cast for her right leg to bring the foot up and to ensure that when she was ready to learn to walk again, her ankle joint would be working properly. However essential it might be for the future, though, this cast proved to be dangerous in the present. When Misti swung her right leg in her bed, she often hit her unprotected left leg with the heavy cast, leaving it looking black and blue and very painful.

Once Misti had her own wheelchair and was sitting up on a regular basis, she was ready for occupational therapy. Each morning, I wheeled her to the occupational therapy room down the hall, where we worked with Terry, a patient and very jolly person. By this time, Misti's eyes were open and she seemed to be staring straight ahead. Terry wanted to find out whether she could see and follow motion. Terry's test for this involved several brightly colored balloons, which she threw toward Misti one by one. The first day, Misti did not blink, indicating she did not see the balloons. However, when the balloons gently hit her, she brought her right hand up as though trying to push them away from her face. As the days passed, we began to realize that she could in fact see the balloons coming, but that her response was slow. Thereafter, each day we tried the same thing, and each day her response got faster. I tried the same thing with Misti back in her room between therapies. Everyone—the nurses, the therapists, and me—continued to encourage her to keep her eyes open, to try to stay awake, but sometimes, fatigue just got the better of her, and she had to nap.

Swallow therapy was frustrating because Misti did not seem to be able to control her mouth very much. At the beginning, she could not swallow at all. In fact, she couldn't even close her mouth completely, and saliva ran from her mouth and had to be wiped away. We would have to work on this; learning how to keep her mouth closed would be an important step toward talking and eating.

The rehab specialists had emphasized that stimulation of all the senses was important for recovering coma patients. Fascinated, I watched as the staff brought televisions, tape players, and radios into the rooms of the patients on Unit 700, patiently, ingeniously trying to find the sound key to breaking through the coma. I was heartened when one young man started singing along with *Sesame Street*. It was his first response to anything, and I hoped that it would be the harbinger of greater recovery. I noticed that when a tape player was brought into the bed with Misti and her favorite tapes were played, she seemed to be moving to the music, but when I reported this, Dr. Audieh explained that a lot of Misti's movements at this point were involuntary, and that she was not necessarily beating time with the music. This was a little discouraging, but as they kept telling us, the brain recovers very unevenly, with involuntary reflexes coming back faster than voluntary movement, and we would have to accept that. At one of the meetings, we had been asked about Misti's favorite television shows, and Misti was now back to listening to, if not watching, her soap operas each day. I would also put the phone receiver next to Misti's ear when friends, family, or Max called.

Now I decided that it was time to expand her world a bit more. I tried to bring something new each day for her to smell, hoping that she would respond. One day I stopped in at a local pizza shop, where I picked up a piece of her favorite food, bringing it into the room and explaining to her that the aroma she was smelling was indeed pizza. Later, I reflected that this might have been frustrating: Imagine being hungry, smelling pizza, and not being able to eat it! I did the same thing with other forms of fast food and their distinctive odors.

I kept thinking about the need to bring familiar odors into Misti's life and thought about the fragrance of flowers, only to be stopped by the realization that, despite the coma, Misti's allergies to grass, trees, and flowers were probably still quite active. One night, I sat down to write to the headmaster at Mercersburg Academy, asking him to have the girls send samples of their colognes, each bottle marked with the name of its owner. My hope was that Misti would be able to connect the different fragrances with the memories of school and her friends. One day not long after, Nurse Betty told me that a box had arrived for me. I rushed to open it, chattering to Misti about what great treasure it might hold. Mercersburg Academy had come through again: The well-padded package was full of cologne bottles, each labeled with a name, many with notes informing me what to tell Misti as I let her smell them. This truly was a treasure, I realized. Many of the bottles had pictures taped to them as well, so I could describe the owner to Misti. As I removed the pictures to mount them on the board, I showed each to Misti, telling her that Kim was sending her love or that Mark had said hello. Spraying the cologne into the air directly in front of her, I explained to her that the lovely smell was Odette, who had just walked into the room. As I talked, I kept praying, "Please let this work; it has to work; she will start to laugh and talk to us any day now."

The teachers and students at Mercersburg seemed determined to keep in touch. In addition to daily cards from family members, every week or so we received batches of letters, cards, and tapes from the Academy. One teacher had the kids spend some time writing to Misti, telling her what was going on in the class and offering hopes for her speedy return. The students, balanced between adolescent awkwardness and adult concern, tried to come up with encouraging things to say to a classmate who had had very bad luck. In their cards and their voices, we could read both their concern and their fear.

Each morning, I fought commuter traffic to get to the Rehab between 7:00 and 7:30 A.M. I would greet Misti, then wash her face for her and freshen her mouth with lemon swabs, since we really couldn't brush her teeth yet. In the beginning, I would help the nurse on duty dress Misti, but before long, I was dressing her myself. I brushed and styled Misti's hair every day, often using a scarf to cover the top, but allowing her beautiful long brown hair to cascade down over her shoulders. I also put a light pink shade of lipstick on her mouth, telling her what I was doing and how nice she looked. I didn't know if I was getting through, but I reasoned that it couldn't hurt. Misti had always been a lovely girl and was very particular about her grooming. I wanted to make sure that she felt as comfortable and attractive—as much like her old self—as possible.

Though the days at the Rehab were long and exhausting, I was convinced that my being with Misti was very important. Some of the patients had no visitors, no one to say that they preferred Beethoven to Bach or always watched *Jeopardy*, and their progress seemed slower than those whose families or friends were able to spend time at the rehab on a regular basis. At the very least, by being there I could make sure that Misti got all of the therapy time for which she was scheduled. Since I was able to get Misti to the therapy rooms before each session, valuable time was not lost in waiting for a volunteer to transport her or for the therapist to set things up. In fact, before long I was making myself useful by taking the departing patient back to his or her room and bringing the next one on the schedule down to the therapy room. I was also able to make sure that small things were attended to quickly. If Misti was agitated for some reason, or if she seemed exhausted or feverish, or if the linen needed changing, I could let someone know immediately. As time went on and the nurses and I became more comfortable with each other, I would often take care of the problem myself. Soon, I was getting Misti showered on the nights it wasn't officially on her schedule.

I looked forward to the weekends, which was generally when Harry could come up and spend a few days. Sometimes he was able to get there by Wednesday night and spend the weekend and on through Tuesday morning; other times, he could stay only Saturday and Sunday. I knew it was good for Harry and Misti to spend time together, and for me to be reminded that I had a partner in this endeavor. In addition to raising my spirits and helping me attend to Misti's needs, Harry was also creative, able to make games out of tedious therapy exercises. One particular Friday found the Morningstar family sitting in the occupational therapy room, batting balloons back and forth—a game we hadn't played since Misti was a baby. When Harry missed catching a balloon, Terry and I started to laugh. Suddenly, we all became aware that Misti was laughing, too. This was very encouraging. Though I thought I heard her make a sound at the same time—perhaps because I wanted so badly to hear her voice again—Terry told me that this was just wishful thinking. However, there was no denying that the right side of Misti's mouth did curl into a smile, and that felt like a small victory.

Each weekend, Harry and I and whoever was visiting worked with Misti to try to get her to keep her eyes open. "Wake up, pretty girl," we'd say. "Open your eyes now, Misti." Or, "Misti, just look at what Daddy's brought you—with both eyes, Princess." Misti seemed to be trying harder to hold her eyes open, and the right one seemed to open much more than the left. When Max and his father arrived the third weekend, they were ecstatic at this change, and even more so when we told them about the balloon game and Misti's smile.

By Monday, Misti was always tired from the weekend's activity and attention; once her guests were gone, she made it clear that she wanted to sleep. Her eyes just wouldn't stay open. I worried that we were pushing her too hard, but I kept remembering that the doctors had said that the longer she stayed in the coma, the worse her prognosis. However much I shared her exhaustion, I also knew that the therapy must be continued. For recovery to take place, it's important to keep building on small pieces of progress.

One day, her right hand reached for the top of her head, where the hair was now standing straight up in a flat-top style. Though she seemed to recognize that something was wrong with the top of her head, she was obviously fascinated and kept trying to feel this new sensation again. When Mr. Burgin saw this on one of his visits, he said he was certain that when Misti returned to Mercersburg, she would set the new style, and everyone would soon be wearing flat-top buzz cuts!

As I watched her slow but definite progress, I was reminded of Misti as a baby, trying new things, touching everything to see how it felt, putting everything in her mouth to test its taste. I guessed that this resemblance made a certain amount of sense. All of the reading I was doing told me that recovery from coma involves the reeducation of the brain, persuading one parcel of nerves to step in and function for another, so I knew I was observing Misti going through a second infancy.

☺

As March rolled on, spring edged closer. Whenever the weather and her therapy schedule permitted, I took Misti out into the courtyard in her wheelchair, putting sunglasses on her to protect her eyes. We also took walks. I would push the wheelchair and talk to her, describing the coming of spring and sharing the family's news. Sometimes I felt myself on the receiving end of pitying looks from staff members who seemed to be trying to tell me that the situation was hopeless.

In fact, after awhile the nurses and doctors began to hint gently that all my hard work was not going to do what I hoped it would. They were also very concerned that my long hours at the Rehab were taking a great toll on me. I should spend more time at the townhouse, they said, or go shopping. I really needed a break or I would have a breakdown or get sick, they insisted. But I could not pull back now. After all, the important thing was not how I was feeling, but how Misti was doing. I wanted to do everything I could to get her back as soon as possible. I had to admit, though, that progress seemed very slow.

By now, I had begun to accept the fact that Misti, exceptional though she had always been, was not going to be the exception to the coma-recovery rule. Yes, Misti was making progress, but very slowly. Only when we made the effort to look back to what she had been capable of doing the previous week in comparison to her current activities could we recognize that Misti's condition was truly improving.

What we needed, I decided, was time-lapse photography, like the kind used in nature specials to show flowers blooming or baby birds hatching. But I didn't need Walt Disney to do this, I realized, since modern technology makes it possible for everyone to make their own movies via the video camera. I asked Harry to bring up our video camera so that I could start videotaping Misti. Not only would this help me remember that progress was being made, but it would be a good record for Misti, who would certainly want to know what had happened to her and whose memory, we had been told, might be impaired in the future. If she got discouraged with the slowness of her progress, we could show her how much improvement there had already been. It took me a while to convince Harry, who at first was reluctant to keep a video record of his injured daughter, but eventually he agreed. Soon he began helping with the taping, and we were able to begin keeping Misti's remarkable video records.

Life in the Rehab was a rollercoaster ride. One day I'd feel down, the next, I'd find my spirits rising again. One day, all of Unit 700 was celebrating the birthday of a patient named Jeff, whose room was two doors down from Misti's. Jeff had been in an accident on Christmas Eve, and now, three months later, he was walking with a cane. It would take hard work, I knew, but maybe Misti could one day do this, too.

Five

As we had been told when Bryn Mawr accepted Misti, every two weeks there were team meetings to discuss her case. The rehab team, which consisted of the head nurse, therapists, doctors, our insurance representative, and Harry and me, would sit down to evaluate Misti's care—the progress she was making, the problems we were encountering, the treatments being tried, the medications she was taking, and the overall concerns of the entire team.

Everyone was invited to offer observations and to put their experiences together to come up with the best possible treatment. Was Misti staying awake longer? Good; now how would we encourage this? She was doing well on the antiseizure medication, but was it making her too groggy? Perhaps we might try something new. Were the casts working, or was it time for new ones? Should we think about removing Misti's nasogastric tube in favor of feedings through a tube directly to her stomach? What were the pros and cons? The concentration that everyone brought to these meetings often allowed news that might otherwise have been overlooked to surface; one staff member might have seen something that the others had missed. The staff always made Harry and me feel like important members of the team. They were interested in our observations because we were the ones most likely to be aware of some small sign of change that the nurses or therapists might miss. They looked to me to tell them if Misti seemed to be more restless than usual, or if she seemed to be in pain, or if some change in the routine had had an unexpected impact.

At the team meetings, we went over and over the different stages of coming out of coma. Most, but not all, recovering coma patients go through every stage, and in the same order. At the Shock Trauma Unit in Bethesda, Misti's condition had been assigned a number on the Glasgow Coma Scale. Numbers were assigned depending on whether she could respond with her eyes, verbally, or with appropriate motor function, and Misti's Glasgow rating had never been higher than nine out of a possible fifteen. However, most rehabilitation facilities used a different scale, one developed at the Rancho Los Amigos Hospital in California, to describe stages of recovery. A coma patient at a Rancho Los Amigos Level of I is only breathing, usually cannot swallow, and makes no response to any kind of stimuli; a patient at Level IV is typically confused and agitated, with some motor function but little control and little ability to make sense of his surroundings. A Level V patient may no longer be agitated but may respond inappropriately to stimuli and may jumble present and past events. A patient at Level VI may still be confused but is able to regain many levels of functioning. At Level VIII, the patient is fully alert and oriented, responds normally and appropriately to a wide variety of stimuli, and has regained significant control over his life. When Misti was first evaluated at Bryn Mawr, she was categorized as being at a Rancho Los Amigos Level of III, meaning that she was breathing on her own, was minimally responsive to specific stimuli, and could follow simple commands, although often in an inconsistent and delayed manner.

After listening to and reading about the descriptions of the various Rancho levels, I developed my own understanding of rehabilitation after brain injury: Since people typically use only ten to fifteen percent of the brain, an advance to a new Rancho level represents getting back another percentage of usable brain. As far as I was concerned, the good news was that the largely unused eighty-five percent of the brain could in many cases be trained to take on the duties of some of the damaged parts. Even when there has been damage to the part of the brain that controls language and some higher level functioning, there is the possibility of retraining the brain, with the help of psychological and educational experts. I understood the idea of physical rehabilitation, but the idea of such cognitive retraining was new to me. As far as I could tell, cognitive retraining would be like a return to early childhood, when a child's brain is soaking up information like a sponge. And it would probably be time-consuming, since the part of the brain being trained was not the part that naturally took up the functions in question. But if the experts were correct about the capacity of the brain for change and development, we had new hope of Misti's general recovery.

At the end of each team meeting, therapy and treatment goals for the next two weeks were planned. The meetings were usually quite heartening because no one was wedded to any particular plan for reasons of ego or seniority and staff members were quite willing to adopt any reasonable suggestion that Harry or I might make despite the fact that we were not rehab specialists. If we reported that Misti was more alert just after breakfast, for instance, or that she was moving one arm or leg a bit more, everyone was excited and happy to put together a plan to use this information to enhance her recovery. When everyone was satisfied that they understood the next steps to be taken and agreed with the plan for doing so, the nurses, doctors, and therapists filed out, leaving us with one or more of the social workers, who stayed behind to talk to us about how we were handling everything. They often asked how Harry was handling the heavy commuting, how Chuck and Cork and their families were doing, and how I felt about not being with my grandchildren, especially the new baby, Victor, who had been born just before

Christmas and who I had not seen in months. My response was that I certainly wished I could be with them more, because the two little ones were changing so fast, but I could not split myself in two. I was only one person and for the time being, this was my life.

As the therapy with the balloons continued, it was becoming obvious even to our inexpert eyes that Misti was trying to bat the balloons back to the person talking to her. When we realized this, Harry and I quickly moved to the opposite side of the room and called Misti to bat the balloons back to us one at a time. By now, Misti's eyes were open most of the time, but it still seemed as though she was more responsive to sounds than to sight. In looking back, I now realize that part of the problem was that she could not see terribly well. Because Misti had been wearing contact lenses for nearsightedness since the age of twelve, we were not used to seeing her in glasses, and so it did not register for a couple of months that she was likely to be having problems with her vision. And since Misti was not able to communicate, she couldn't tell us, nor could we have tested her vision in any dependable manner. If the damage to her brain had adversely affected her vision—which was possible because there had been damage to the occipital lobe of her brain, which takes care of vision—we would not know about it for some time. It would a long while before even Misti could recognize and process her difficulties in seeing.

Meanwhile, other kinds of therapy continued, depending on the particular day's schedule. In occupational therapy, the therapist might show Misti pictures and ask her to look for the bicycle, the house, or the dog, even though she showed almost no sign that she had even heard the request. In speech therapy, the therapist would hold Misti's hand against her own throat to feel the vibrations and against her mouth to feel the breath in hopes that Misti would begin to make sounds of her own. When we started, it was hard to believe that Misti had any idea what was going on. We had to hold on to what we were told: After traumatic brain injury, the brain heals at its own pace. Because Misti was still so tired, we had to schedule a rest period between therapy sessions. She particularly needed to rest up for physical therapy.

At this early point, physical therapy was fairly simple. It often consisted of something elementary, like trying to get Misti to hold up her head and move her right arm as much as possible, with the therapists moving her legs and other arm. Or they might roll her over on the table and get her into a sitting position with her legs hanging down over the side in order to get her torso upright. When someone is mostly paralyzed, I'd learned, independent movement must start from a strong and stabilized torso, so we all tried hard to get Misti used to sitting up. Sitting up was also required for swallow therapy to work, so this exercise served a dual function. Cognitive therapy sessions reminded me a lot of occupational therapy, but I suspected that once Misti had had some success it would be different.

Misti was still getting her meals through a tube, and we'd go back to her room for this, though I always made a point of taking Misti along when I went to the cafeteria to have lunch or dinner. After dinner, I'd usually take Misti for a walk, either inside the Rehab or outside if the weather was nice. Then we'd go back to Misti's room to open the mail that had arrived that day. I would read each card to Misti and talk about the people who sent the cards—who they were and where they lived. After we'd gone through the mail, I'd make a call to Harry or one of the boys, reporting on the day's events so they'd know what was going on and in turn could let our friends and neighbors in Waynesboro know. Then it was off to the shower and back to Misti's room to get her ready for bed. After such a full day, it usually took her very little time to drop off to sleep.

☺

Because Misti could not swallow or eat, toothbrushing had been replaced by the application of lemon-flavored mouth swabs. One day after physical therapy, the usual lemon-swab mouth refresher revealed spots of bright red blood in her mouth, along with a great amount of mucus. Praying hard that Misti would not clamp down on my fingers with her teeth, I forced her tongue up to locate the source of the blood. Almost two months after the accident, Misti was still wearing an orthodontic retainer on the inside of her bottom teeth, and that appliance had broken. A piece of the metal wire had worked its way loose from the retainer and stabbed into the bottom of her tongue. I couldn't recall seeing this before—certainly, this was the first sign of blood that I had seen or anyone had mentioned—and I winced in sympathy. Misti must be in great pain, I knew, but she had had no way to tell us. Moving

47

quickly, I phoned her orthodontist in Waynesboro for advice. This wonderfully kind man immediately said he'd come up and take care of the situation. Then, realizing that he had an office full of patients and would not be able to leave Waynesboro for several hours, he offered to call a dentist friend who had a practice not far from the rehab. I should sit tight and not panic, he said; he would phone his friend and then call me back.

While waiting for his call, I reported the broken appliance to one of the nurses. This proved to be frustrating because the nursing staff were obliged to fill out a formal report. They told me that the rules required that only a doctor or dentist registered with the institution would be allowed to attend to Misti. I knew about insurance concerns and that rules must be obeyed, but I found myself operating on a stronger force: maternal instinct. My daughter, paralyzed and helpless, was suffering, and something had to be done now.

I now wished I had not brought the problem to the attention of the nurses, and I wondered how long we would have to wait. When the phone rang, I leapt to answer it. Misti's orthodontist was on the other end, explaining that he had already talked with the dentist in Paoli and suggesting I phone him also. I decided to use the phone in the lobby so the nurses would not overhear the call. Fortunately, the dentist had already been informed of all the details and readily agreed to come out and cut the appliance from Misti's mouth early that evening. I was grateful, but I realized that I would have to come up with a plan if this was going to happen. Back in Misti's room, the nurses and Dr. Audieh were discussing how to take care of the problem. Finally I was told that in accordance with Bryn Mawr policy, Misti would be transported by ambulance to Paoli Hospital, and the problem would be corrected as soon as this could be arranged. This, I distantly heard them say, would take place sometime in the next two weeks.

My mind spinning with unaccustomed guile, I heard myself telling them that we were expecting a visitor later that afternoon. I was sure that my fib would be my undoing, since I realized that I had not even asked the man what he looked like. I had merely given him directions to Misti's room that would allow him to bypass the nurses' station. "Just act like you know what you are doing and where you are going, and everything will be okay. I will be waiting at her door," I had told him on the phone.

As I waited for this compassionate man to appear, I felt almost totally alone. It did not seem right to ask God's help to carry out something that was not quite honest, though I was sure that I was right to try to take care of the problem immediately. At 5:05 P.M., I drew the draperies on the windows separating Misti's room from the nurses' station and told the staff that Misti was resting. Usually when I did this, the staff made sure not to disturb her, and I hoped that this would be the case today. As the time passed, I realized that I was a bundle of nerves. Could I carry this off? Would we get caught? Quietly, carefully, I moved Misti from the bed to her chair, explaining as I did so what was going to happen. My heart leapt into my mouth as a shadow appeared in the doorway—not a nurse, not now, I thought, please not now—but the shadow turned out to be a man carrying a small black case. The kindness in his face brought great relief, but my heart was still beating uncontrollably and my hands shook. Calmly, quietly, he opened Misti's mouth, cut loose the broken appliance, and removed it. Fortunately, there was very little bleeding from her sore and swollen tongue. As he handed me the wire appliance, I offered to pay him, but he just smiled and said that I should do something for someone else when they needed it. He shook my hand and said, "God bless," and walked out through the door as quietly as he had come in. I looked at Misti and said, with a smile, "Who was that masked man?"

As things turned out, there were really no consequences to my having taken care of the problem myself. My guess is that when the weekend nursing staff came in to check on Misti's mouth and saw that the appliance had been removed, they just crossed the problem off their to-do list. They were probably glad not to have to fill out more forms and deal with more red tape. In any case, no one said anything to me about it. The important thing was that Misti was now out of pain—and in a much shorter period of time than if I'd done nothing.

Misti's immediate problem having been taken care of, I now turned my thoughts to the weekend. Harry would be arriving any time now, as would Max, who drove up to Bryn Mawr each Friday as soon as school was dismissed for the week. Once again, I was struck by how unfair all this was: Max, at seventeen, had given up his weekends, his extracurricular activities, and his social life to be with Misti, and she did not even seem to know when he was here. This was clearly a huge burden on him; he seemed very young to have to make such a great sacrifice, but then, at seventeen, neither he nor Misti should have been suffering this way. They should be dancing, laughing, and going to movies. After Max arrived and took up his usual position of lying in the Bryn Mawr bed beside Misti and stroking her hand, I could only wonder what they might have accomplished together or apart, where their lives might have gone under other circumstances.

Later that evening, for the first time since the accident, Harry and I both seemed to run out of optimism at the same time. At Chesterbrook, we discussed the fact that the situation really seemed to be very little better now than it had been back in Bethesda. Yes, Misti was keeping her eyes open these days, but was she really in there somewhere, with her personality intact? In spite of all we had learned about retraining the brain and various forms of therapy, we had no way to know whether she could in fact recover from this or what recovery would entail. In our many years of marriage, Harry and I had learned to balance ourselves; we very seldom were both down at the same time, so we could usually encourage each other when the situation looked bleak. Now, for the first time since the accident, both of us were having doubts, and though Harry tried hard to tell me that everything would be all right, I felt heavy with despair.

After a sobering Saturday, Sunday dawned clear and bright. Max's parents, Brenda and Anthony, drove up, and knowing that I needed both a break and a lift, Harry and Max offered to keep Misti company so that I could take a walk down the road to attend a church service. I needed the strong arms of a comforting community around me. The church was very pleasant, modern for such a country setting and much smaller than our local church in Waynesboro. The people in the congregation were friendly and welcoming. One particular woman sitting beside me seemed to be jabbering all through the service; at first, I thought she might have a hearing problem, because the sounds she made were loud enough to be heard over most of the service. After the benediction, however, she turned to me and explained that she had the gift of speaking in tongues. I was not sure exactly what this meant and drifted away from her.

I talked to several people who had stopped to say hello and invite me to come back for other services. Some even asked if they could visit Misti during the week, and I gratefully accepted their offers. The stimulation would be good for Misti, and despite phone calls and intermittent visits from the family, I was extremely lonely during the week. The minister, too, said that he would come to the Rehab and offered to contact our pastor in Waynesboro and let him know how Misti and I were doing.

As I arrived back at Bryn Mawr, I saw that Max had Misti propped up almost in a standing position, which had upset the nurse on duty greatly. She was pointing out to him that though he was only trying to help, Misti could in fact be injured if handled improperly. Misti's head hung to her left shoulder and only one eye was open; her arms were limp, and her legs seemed unable to hold up even her small amount of weight. Her appearance brought to mind a well-loved rag doll from my youth. As the nurses lowered her carefully into the bed she seemed very confused; one eye remained open while the other fluttered uncontrollably. As usual after any exertion, she was very tired and rested for several hours, unable to make any response. When Max left, later in the day, it was easy to tell that he felt defeated and frustrated at his inability to help. I did not like to see him make the long drive home in this depressed mental state, but there was no way around it since he had to be back for school the next day.

That evening, after dinner with friends from Harrisburg, Harry and I went back to the Rehab to get Misti ready for bed. The phone was ringing as I walked into her room; when I picked it up, I found myself talking to a friend of Misti's who had moved to Texas several months before. Although she had heard that Misti had been in an accident, she had no idea of how serious it was or of Misti's condition. As I explained the situation to her, sobs rocked the long-distance lines from Texas to Pennsylvania. When she had regained some of her composure, I put the phone to Misti's ear so she could talk to her. Later, she gave me a number for Misti to call her "when she is better."

On St. Patrick's Day, I made a point of digging out Misti's old green William and Mary University sweat shirt and pants, to try to cheer Misti—and myself—up. Her outfit was bright, cheerful, seasonable, and most important, familiar. If she were to come out of the coma, she would not panic at being clad in clothing she'd never seen before. In spite of Misti's cheerful attire and the festive attitude of the staff at the Rehab, however, it was a hard day. Since St. Patrick's Day was also Chuck's birthday, the day had always been one of family celebration. That night, Chuck called and told me he had just gotten back from Williamsburg with Teresa and the children. I was glad he had been able to continue on with his life. He explained that he was now attending sales seminars and working the business just as though I was there. This made me feel good in some ways; I was glad that he and Cork had been able to go on with their lives. But I also felt lonely. This would be the first birthday that I would not bake him a cake and have some kind of celebration, even if it was just having the family for dinner. And though I spoke with him daily, I was beginning to feel that I hadn't actually had a regular conversation with Harry in weeks. Easter would soon be here; what would I be doing then? I usually made a big fuss for family holidays, especially with the grandchildren. Would life ever get back to normal?

☉

Harry's brother Dave and his wife Beck made the first of what would be semimonthly visits the next weekend, and as always, they were tremendously comforting and helpful. They always seemed to be there at just the right moment; I don't know what we would have done without them. They took great care of Harry and me without making a big fuss about it. They didn't lecture or argue, or, like the well-meaning Bryn Mawr social workers, say, "You must get away and watch out for your own health." Instead, they showed up and said and did the things that made it possible for us to relax. For instance, on that weekend they announced that they wanted to visit a particular bookstore in Philadelphia that had gotten a lot of publicity recently, and since Max had arrived to keep Misti company, they insisted that we go along.

This trip was the first time I had really been out in public since the accident, and I had almost forgotten that there was a world beyond the Rehab. In Center City Philadelphia, we saw a lot of street kids with long, bedraggled hair and dirty clothes who were certainly unconcerned about and in some cases totally unaware that they were lucky enough to be alive and well. It was clear to me that these kids were drunk or high; many still carried the previous night's bottle in a brown bag. As I watched them, tears rolled down my face. I looked up to God and asked, "Why Misti? Why not one of these kids? What will they ever amount to anyway? Would the world be changed if they all disappeared tonight?" Then a verse from an early childhood song came to my mind: "Red and yellow, black and white, they are precious in his sight. Jesus loves the little children of the world." These were some of his children also, just as important to him as Misti or any of her classmates. Suddenly, I was ashamed of myself.

When we arrived back at the Rehab, refreshed after our break, Max was positively glowing. Almost tripping over the words in his pride, he told us that while we were away, Misti had turned over from her back to her stomach, on her own. This represented definite progress, and when Max left to drive home at the end of the weekend, I was much less worried about his making the drive alone and depressed.

As therapy of all kinds continued, Misti began to move more. Though the nurses, doctors, and therapists told us this was a good sign, the new movement of her arms and legs was accompanied by increasing agitation. She became restless and often downright uncooperative, refusing to help with transfers from bed to wheelchair, and fighting us and the nursing staff when we tried to change her clothes. She had also begun to pull on her feeding tube, which she found irritating. If she were successful in pulling the tube out, not only would it be necessary to reinsert it, which would require X-rays to make sure that the position was correct, but the feedings that she needed to gain back the weight she had lost would be interrupted. Once again, Misti was taking one step forward, only to fall back again. She had also become recalcitrant with the therapists as they went about their exercises. This was discouraging, even though we had been told that it meant that Misti's brain had started to recover and was beginning to reactivate. Though this stage of agitation passed in time, it was hard not to take personally. This was when I really began to appreciate how good the nursing at Bryn Mawr was. I marveled as I watched Peggy, Linda, and Betty treat Misti with endless good humor and patience, even when she was trying to pull out her nasogastric tube or was making it difficult to transfer her to a wheelchair, and I reminded myself that there was a reason that patience is one of the cardinal virtues.

In late March, after nearly a month of brutal commuting, Harry was able to spend an entire week with me at Bryn Mawr. By this time, the worst of Misti's agitation seemed to have passed. Having heard from me and witnessed for himself on weekends how difficult Misti could be, Harry was delighted to see that she had begun to quiet down some. That week marked other changes as well: Dr. Audieh made the decision to change Misti's anti-seizure medication from Dilantin to Tegretol, a milder medication we hoped would allow her to be more alert and perhaps need less sleep. The change from one medication to another, however, proved to be a little more momentous than we expected, and Misti got violently ill, suddenly throwing up on anything and anyone. In our traditional household, I had always been the one to take care of the children when they were sick, but this occasion found Harry pitching right in and doing whatever had to be done. His only comment was, "I just hope this will help her."

This whole experience was so hard on Harry, I thought, as I watched him care for Misti. When it came to raising Chuck and Cork, Harry was always on solid ground: He taught them everything he knew about camping and hunting and made sure they had always had the proper instructions before handling guns and other outdoors equipment. And of course, he had worked with them in the business. Very matter-of-fact with the boys, he had always been a little awed when it came to his daughter. He was immensely proud of her, and even though she was adopted, his chest swelled visibly whenever anyone said, "Misti looks like her father." But if he ceded me the day-to-day activities of child care, Harry excelled as a father in other ways. For instance, he was an outstanding planner. He had always been careful to make sure that in addition to our regular medical insurance, we had a second insurance policy to cover anything over a million dollars. I was immensely thankful that he had always been so meticulous about these things; I am more scattered, and I knew how badly things might have gone had it been my responsibility to plan for such emergencies. Now, as I watched his tender care of Misti, I was so thankful we had met; over the years, we had made a great team, and I was able to reassure myself that together we would conquer even this.

Since Max stayed with me at Chesterbrook on weekends if his parents did not come up to visit, we had many opportunities to talk. One night, we found ourselves discussing Misti's adoption. As I explained to Max, adopting a child was complicated, especially when a couple already had children. For instance, in our home state of Pennsylvania, where Harry and I originally applied to adopt a daughter, we were told that our names would be near the bottom of a lengthy waiting list. At the time, Maryland's adoption laws were a bit more liberal than Pennsylvania's, and Harry and I decided to apply there. We went down to Hagerstown, which was only about fifteen miles south of Waynesboro but across the Maryland state line, and talked to officials in the welfare office there.

We filled out lengthy applications, then awaited the necessary interviews and endless questions. In fairly short order, we were assigned a social worker, a tall, very businesslike and professional woman named Mary Broadwater, whose job was to judge which of the many families who were applying to adopt could be entrusted with a priceless life. Nature had failed to give us a daughter, but Mrs. Broadwater had it in her power to correct that—if she deemed us suitable. She was an extremely no-nonsense sort of person and clearly took her responsibilities seriously; I felt that she couldn't be kidded or fooled, that she could see through any attempts to cover things up. Never once during the time we worked with her did she share any personal details, such as whether she herself had children or knew what it was like to long for a child. Yet, as soon as I met her I had an uncanny sense that she was someone who would see how very much we wanted to give a good home to a daughter, someone who would work very hard to help us add a little girl to our family.

Over several months' time she made a number of visits to our home to look it—and us—over. She talked to me and to Harry, as well as to Chuck and Cork, separately and together, and in all combinations. Some of her questions, such as what attracted Harry to me in the first place or how we worked together as a team to raise our children, seemed nosy, but it made sense that Mrs. Broadwater needed to know how stable our marriage and family values were.

Because we already had two children, we knew we were facing great odds in trying to adopt an infant; healthy infants usually went to childless couples. Mrs. Broadwater told us that our chances of adopting would be better if we were willing to take a child who was difficult to place—an older child, for instance, or a handicapped child. We really felt we'd do better with a baby, we said, though we were willing to take a child up to five years old or so, and we were certainly willing to consider adopting a handicapped child. When we said this, Mrs. Broadwater asked us what kind of handicap we could handle. We had to be very clear on this, since a child was not merchandise to be returned to the store if it did not suit us after a while. Quite honestly, said Harry, he didn't think he could do a good job of raising a retarded child; twelve years of parenthood had taught him that his expectations for his children tended to be high. For my part, I said, I'd have a hard time with a blind child, because a sense of the visually beautiful—color, patterns, light, and darkness—was so important to me. What about a child born without arms or legs, we were asked, since the nation had recently seen the birth of such children due to the thalidomide tragedy. This, we felt, would not be a problem, since a child so challenged would just need us more.

After the interviews and inspections, Mrs. Broadwater only said that perhaps we would be meeting again. Despite the lack of any firm commitment—and the fact that we were running against a deadline, since Harry was about to turn thirty-five, the cut-off age for adoptive fathers—I had a feeling that we would indeed get a daughter, an unshakable belief that it would be only a matter of time, of waiting patiently, before we had a little girl.

About seven months later, we received a call from Mrs. Broadwater telling us that the state of Maryland had a child for us. Breathlessly, we asked if the child had a birth defect, only to hear Mrs. Broadwater say that, although she really couldn't talk about it over the phone, the baby did have a handicap and it was "rather funny." Harry and I were stunned to hear this levity; this just didn't sound like the Mrs. Broadwater we had come to know. When we saw her the next day, she immediately apologized for her choice of words, saying that she'd never meant to make fun of so serious a subject, but the fact of the matter was that the baby girl had been born with six toes on each foot. Harry blurted out, "That's got to be our daughter," and then we all burst into laughter. Now we realized why Mrs. Broadwater had said the baby's handicap was funny. In the course of the long examination process, we'd told Mrs. Broadwater that Harry had been born with six fingers on his hands. Clearly, we all recognized, Misti was meant to be a Morningstar.

At five weeks, Misti was a beautiful baby, with dark eyes and soft shiny hair. Mrs. Broadwater was able to tell us little of her biological parents, only that both were professionals, unmarried, that they had split up just prior to the mother discovering that she was pregnant. According to the agency's social workers, the mother was very practical and businesslike, but had also done a lot of soul searching before deciding to continue the pregnancy and put the baby up for adoption. We were told that the father was quite attractive, with dark eyes and dark curly hair, and that he had offered to marry the mother once he learned that the child was on the way. But the mother had refused because, she said, it was "better not to compound an error and make three lives miserable." For all her resolve, however, it had taken quite some time for the mother to bring herself to sign the necessary papers freeing the baby for adoption, and during that time, the baby had remained in the hospital. While the father knew that he had a daughter and had insisted on seeing her, the mother refused to learn the sex of the baby. Finally, she called the agency's social workers late one evening and told them that if they brought the necessary papers over immediately, she would sign them. Mrs. Broadwater told us that we must never refer to Misti's mother derogatorily, and I remember wondering how anyone could feel anything but compassion for a woman who had gone through childbirth alone and had been unselfish enough to give up her firstborn in order to provide her with a family and a full life.

As I looked back over our lives and hers, I was pleased that Misti had grown up with so much self-confidence. I distinctly remembered the first day I took her to nursery school, her hand clasped firmly in mine. We walked up to the teacher, who said, "Good morning, my name is Mrs. Zimmerman, and I'm your teacher. Who are you and what is special about you?" Misti looked into the face of this stranger and strongly replied, "I'm Misti Morningstar, and I'm adopted." A few weeks later the teacher would call and tell me that Misti's forthright explanation of her origins had the other kids in the class feeling neglected; even her own daughter cried because she had not been "chosen" like Misti and two of the other children in the class. Of course, Misti was not trying to be cruel. Taking her cue from what we told her at home, she had merely explained to her classmates that being adopted meant that you had been selected and not just expected. Misti felt that being adopted was special because we always told her how special she was to us. And it was not just Harry and me who said so; Chuck and Cork always let her know that all our lives had changed for the better because she was a part of our family.

Because we had heard from other families who had adopted that it would be a traumatic blow were Misti to find out as a teenager that she been adopted, we chose to tell her from the very beginning. And to make everyone comfortable with the idea of adoption, we used the word a lot and made adoption an everyday affair, adopting pets, dolls, and anything else special that we wanted to be part of our family. Over the years, we adopted a dog, even giving him the fancy name of "Paul Tillmington Morningstar, III" to offset his very plain looks; we adopted chocolate bunnies from the kids' Easter baskets and Cabbage Patch kids, who came with their own adoption papers; we even adopted an alligator named George.

Max broke into my happy reverie on Misti's adoption with the news that a few days before the accident, Misti had told him that she wanted to try to find her biological mother. She had asked him not to tell Harry or me since she was going to talk to us about it when we returned from the Caribbean. We had always let her know that if she ever wanted to find her parents, we would do anything we could to help her, but secretly, I hoped that she would never want to. Although I had carefully recorded all the facts I had been given in order to make the task as easy as possible, in my heart of hearts, I wasn't sure I would be unselfish enough to share the honor of being Misti's mother with anyone else. At the same time, I knew that Misti was an intelligent child and would probably want to seek out her other family, her heritage. Now, in speaking with Max, I felt a twinge of guilt about not having pursued the subject with Misti. Maybe now she would never have an opportunity to learn about her biological parents.

Six

After Misti had been at Bryn Mawr Rehab for a month or so, Dr. Audieh decided that the time had come to remove her nasogastric tube and install a feeding tube directly into her stomach. After brain injury that interferes with swallowing and eating, it is common practice to install a nasogastric tube in order to feed the patient. The theory is that if recovery is quick, the patient will not have to have surgery in order to get nourishment. However, there are drawbacks as well: The patient has the disfigurement of a tube running out of his or her nose; if the tube gets dislodged, the patient runs the risk of infection and further weakness; further, the longer the nasogastric tube stays in place, the greater the chance of irritation of delicate tissues in the nose and throat. In her agitation Misti had been pulling at her nasogastric tube, resulting in infections and in irritation, and since recovery of eating and swallowing would clearly require further therapy, Dr. Audieh made the arrangements for her to be taken by ambulance to Paoli Memorial Hospital, where the surgery would be done.

At Paoli, an endoscope was inserted into Misti's mouth and threaded down her esophagus and to her stomach. Using the scope, the surgeon made an incision in Misti's abdomen and inserted a feeding tube. With remarkably little fuss or loss of blood, Misti would now have a much easier time of being fed, with less irritation and much improvement to her general appearance.

After the placement of the stomach tube, Misti's progress seemed to speed up. Although her liquid meals needed a good hour to settle, the consistent nourishment she was getting gave her additional strength, and her movements increased. Even her left leg, which, like her left arm, had been nearly motionless since the accident, began to move a bit, especially after she began water therapy.

When Harry and I had first been investigating rehab facilities, we learned that Bryn Mawr Rehab was in the process of installing a large heated pool for patients. Stroke patients, brain injured patients, and patients who'd been in accidents would all benefit from exercise in the heated water, which offered much more resistance than air. In addition, the water gave buoyancy, which meant that patients who needed wheel-chairs on land could often walk in the pool. Physical therapists worked individually with patients, all of whom wore flotation devices and many of whom had to be lowered into the pool in special chairs.

Even though I'd watched the therapists work with patients from Unit 700, I was a bit surprised when it was time for Misti to start this form of therapy because she still seemed rather unresponsive. But, Misti loved water therapy. She had always been a water baby, and as a toddler, she'd learned to swim before she'd learned to walk. Her flexible feeding tube could be folded inside her bathing suit, and since it had a valve that could be shut to keep water out, there was no danger that she'd pick up an infection. Once she was in the pool, she was able to move with much less effort, and this increased mobility carried over into regular physical therapy as well.

Not long after she'd started water exercise, Misti startled us all by picking her nearly useless left arm up with her right hand and moving it. This was short-lived, though, and she soon began to ignore that arm as well as all our pleas that she try to move it. Fortunately, resourceful Harry stepped in before Misti got too entrenched in her refusal. He brought in several rubber Koosh balls with their soft rubber hair strands and announced that the unusual balls were left-handed balls and could only be played with by the left hand.

Most of the time, we made great efforts to keep Misti's hands palm side down on the tray of her wheelchair, since they tended to curl into awkward claws if they were placed palm up. In order to get her to begin to move and use her left hand, however, we'd place her hands palm up and drop the Koosh balls into her hands. Patiently, hour after hour, Harry would talk to her: "Look, Misti, I'm throwing a ball into your right hand. Be sure to catch it. Now I'm throwing a ball into your left hand, Misti. Remember, that's a left-handed ball, so you can't catch it with your right hand, only the left." Misti seemed fascinated by the texture of the Kooshes and readily accepted the idea of right-handed and left-handed balls. Within a few days, she began to move both hands in order to play with the balls, making real progress toward recovering some left-side movement.

Now a bit more alert, Misti clearly enjoyed having Harry around, and I shed some of my sense of loneliness for the first time in weeks. Then it was time for Harry to go back to Waynesboro and the challenge of starting a real estate development project there. As always, it was hard to see him go.

Larry Jones, the chaplain from Mercersburg Academy, had always been one of Misti's favorite people and had visited her at the STU in Bethesda. He now began coming up to the Rehab from time to time to see Misti, telling her about the school, her classes, friends, how much everyone there missed her—though at the beginning, it was never clear whether Misti could see him or recognize his voice. On one particular day, however, Mr. Jones and I both realized that she knew he was there. As he held her hand, she tried to raise his hand to feel the short stubby hair on top of her head. It was as if she was trying to share with him part of her world. After Mr. Jones's visit, we began to have other visitors from the Academy, usually in the company of Mr. Needham. Despite what they had been told about brain trauma, the students were often very upset to see Misti's condition, though they always tried to be brave and cheerful while they were in her room.

As we moved into April, Misti started to move more and more and her reactions and movements seemed to be speeding up—partly due to brain recovery and partly, we assumed, due to the switch in antiseizure medication. But this step forward, too, had its drawbacks. One day, while a nurse was leaning over her and tending to her needs, Misti whipped her head around quickly and bit her hard enough to draw blood. It happened so quickly that I was reminded of George, the baby alligator we had adopted and nursed back to health one summer. When my brother brought the ailing George to us—he was a school teacher and had had the alligator in his classroom—he told us we would have to feed him raw hamburger by opening his mouth and pushing the meat as far back as we could and then holding his mouth shut until he swallowed. As the regimen of hamburger and warm summer sunshine did its work, George began to get stronger. After a few weeks he graduated to dead minnows, and a few weeks later he was doing his own hunting. By the end of summer, he had grown about eight inches longer and was so quick that he had become dangerous, lashing out with his razor-sharp teeth at anyone and anything that came near him. Needless to say, when fall arrived, George had to be moved from our backyard to a new and safer home.

I told Misti the story of George and how he bit and how much it would hurt people if she ever did it again, but to no avail. All the talking in the world was not enough to stop Misti, who had learned to do something new and was not about to stop biting just because we told her to. The rest of the week offered more proof, if we needed it, that the brain recovering from injury heals in its own way, at its own pace.

One afternoon, Mr. Needham brought a van full of Misti's school-mates from Mercersburg Academy to visit. After Mr. Needham and I exchanged hellos, I explained that Misti had begun biting people and might bite one of her visitors if they were not exceedingly careful. He assured me that Misti would never bite him. Then, as usual, he went in to see her on his own, so he could explain to the day's batch of students, many of whom had not visited before, what to expect before they went in. He walked toward the wheelchair and greeted Misti affectionately. Taking her hand in his, he glanced toward me as if to say that I had to be wrong; Misti would never hurt him. And in fact, at the moment, Misti seemed very loving: She had dropped her head and with his hand at her cheek was moving ever so slowly, as though she did indeed recognize her favorite teacher. Then, as Mr. Needham's hand brushed Misti's cheek in a tender gesture, she moved very quickly and, without warning, sank her teeth into his hand.

Outside in the hallway, tears filled his eyes as he told the students that, for their own safety, they had to keep their distance from Misti when they went in to visit. He explained the situation in detail—that she might bite them hard enough to draw blood. The kids found it very hard to believe that the classmate they remembered could do such a horrible thing, but they could also see the wound on Mr. Needham's hand. One of the girls cried so hard that she was unable to go into the room; another tried to tough it out but collapsed as she walked through the door.

By this time, I had become so accustomed to the way Misti looked that I could see only improvement from the months before. But after the kids left, I deliberately stepped back and looked at Misti with their eyes. It was not surprising that, seeing her for the first time since the accident, some of her schoolmates had had such violent responses. If it was not supported by the strap connected to the halo on her wheelchair, Misti's head flopped to one side; her mouth hung open, letting spittle drop down over her clothes, like an infant. If her twisted arms and legs were not to dangle awkwardly, we had to keep putting them back into the proper holders on the wheelchair. Nor was Misti the same slim and shapely girl she had always been. After several months of inactivity, the middle of her body had begun to thicken from lack of exercise. It was now impossible to tell that for fourteen years she had been a dancer.

When Max and Harry arrived for the weekend the nurses explained to them, too, that Misti was now biting and they should be careful, but both were that sure she would not, could not, bite them. How wrong their assumptions turned out to be. As she recovered from the coma, our sweet-natured daughter was behaving like a wild animal: She would lie very still, but when anyone got near, she attacked without warning, biting the nearest hand, arm, leg. No amount of reasoning with her helped. When we expressed concern and chagrin, Dr. Audieh explained that Misti was not really trying to bite anyone, but her mind was fighting to get out of the coma, to make contact in any way possible. Though this was not unprecedented, especially in patients at a Rancho Los Amigos Level of III, the situation could be serious if it continued for too long. Further, since her bites had drawn blood on a few people, she had to be tested for HIV. At the time, the letters HIV meant nothing to me. Dr. Audieh explained that the Rehab had a responsibility to check for AIDS. As unlikely as it might seem, Misti might have been exposed to the virus and, thus, might be exposing others through her biting. At this, my mind slid into panic mode: Didn't we already have enough to worry about? Could something as bad as AIDS really happen to Misti? Fortunately, this threat passed.

Though it had been several months since the accident, cards and flowers were still arriving daily from home. In fact, now there were several scrapbooks of cards on the book shelf in her room. Each day, after the mail arrived, I read the cards and letters to Misti, then punched holes in the cards and put them in a notebook, noting the date and the sender's return address on the back for future reference. On quiet days, when I had run out of news from home and the Academy and reminiscences and family stories, I reread the cards to Misti, thinking as I did that someday I would have to sit down and write each of these people to let them know how much their messages had meant to me and to Misti.

One day as I was reading the cards, I glanced across the Bryn Mawr bed to share a smile with Misti and was stunned to see that she was snapping the fingers on her right hand. The gesture made no sound, but she seemed to be trying to get my attention. My heart in my throat, I pressed the call bell for Peggy, who was in the room in only seconds. Tears came to her eyes as she saw Misti's clicking fingers. Another sign of improvement. Though it might have been involuntary movement, and thus of no meaning, it seemed to me more likely that Misti was really trying to get my attention, that she was definitely in there, fighting to get out!

Later that week, Chuck and Teresa came up for a visit, bringing their daughter, Valera, and Misti's two grandmothers. Harry's mother always seemed to be able to roll with the punches, but it was hard for her to see Misti in this state. It was even harder for my mother, who hadn't seen Misti since the accident. With all her problems at home taking care of my ailing father, this was the first time she had been able to arrange for someone to stay with him so she could take a day off and visit Misti. Emotionally and physically exhausted, and missing the support she'd always gotten from my previously strong father, she was horrified by the sight of her beloved granddaughter in a large "dog box" with half of her face expressionless. Once outside Misti's room, she cried and asked, "Why Misti?" I certainly knew how she felt, but after a couple of months spent dealing with shock trauma units, rehab facilities, and lots of doctors and nurses, I was able to give her my philosophy on the fairness and unfairness of life. "Why not Misti?" I said. "Perhaps God felt that we are more able to handle the devastating results of such an accident than some other parents." She was not at all happy to hear this, but at least at the moment, I believed what I'd just said. After all, some mothers can't handle a child needing stitches; some even go into shock at the sight of blood. And some fathers just turn their backs and walk away from anything they cannot handle. Though neither of us was having an easy time of it, Harry and I were in fact able to cope with the situation, to keep going even when events were very discouraging.

Not long after, Uncle Ora and Aunt Goldie came up to keep me company and help with Misti's therapy if they could. Most visitors came to the Rehab because that was where I spent the bulk of my time, so I especially appreciated people like Ora and Goldie, who would spend the night with me. Even though I got home each night exhausted, sleep never came easy, and the nights were long and very lonely. In fact, though I was surrounded by people all day, in some ways I had never felt so alone in my life. Since I left the town house so early in the morning, I seldom saw any of the neighbors, and by the time I returned at night, they had all settled into their evenings with their families. I had thought about going next door and introducing myself, but I shied away from letting anyone know that I was so alone. I wrestled with this dilemma constantly; after I'd spoken to Harry or the boys at the end of the day, I was acutely aware of my loneliness. When we returned to the house that night, Aunt Goldie and Uncle Ora reminded me that this wasn't Waynesboro, where I knew everyone and everyone knew me; we were close to a big city, and perhaps I should just keep to myself. After all, Uncle Ora said, maybe it would not be much longer before Misti recovered. But in my heart, I knew that we were nowhere near out of the woods.

The next day, Aunt Goldie and Uncle Ora got an unvarnished view of just how distressing life in a rehab facility for the brain injured can be. As we entered Misti's room, we were nearly overcome by an unmistakable smell. Misti had come down with diarrhea and was covered in her own feces. She would have to be showered and changed, and the bed completely scrubbed down. With Peggy's help, I moved Misti onto a stretcher and got the process started, but by the time she was cleaned up, both Peggy and I were covered with the mess. Uncle Ora and Aunt Goldie quickly offered to run out and get me clean clothes, but before they had the chance to leave, Misti did a repeat performance. Goldie would have to bring several changes for me, since the odds were that this would happen again today. Realizing this was the case, Goldie smiled and I started to laugh; if I hadn't laughed, I might have cried, and I knew that if I started to cry, I might never be able to stop.

Later that day, after Goldie and Ora left to go home, I started to wonder in exhaustion if God might have forgotten that we still existed. But when the mail arrived, I was reassured that there was no way he could forget; the prayer chains were still going strong, from coast to coast, even continent to continent. If anything, I thought, God might be getting tired of hearing from all these people about the same matter. Well, I thought, it serves him right; maybe he would soon decide to make Misti well so that everyone would stop bugging him and let him get on to something else.

Arriving home that night with my plastic bag of smelly clothing, already dead tired, I faced another problem: Since the townhouse did not have a washing machine, and I hadn't had a chance to use the laundry facilities at the Rehab, I would have to wash out each piece of soiled clothing by hand in the bath tub. My black mood was back. Sincerely, I wondered, could God have forgotten about us? On the way to the Rehab the next morning, I wound down the window and screamed, "God, there are other people in the world. Can't you give some of life's problems to a few others? Why keep giving it all to me?"

Fortunately, however, the situation was a little better than the previous day; Misti had not had another attack of diarrhea. She had, however, managed to pull the cast on her left arm down from the elbow to her forearm, and her hand was completely hidden inside the white hard plaster. The cast would have to be removed and a new one put on. Since she was still biting anyone who could get near, this would prove to be a major task in itself. After much consultation with the staff, Misti was put into the wheelchair and her head tied with a restraint; as long as no one got near her head, the chances of being bitten were lessened. All the activity with the cast tired Misti out, and when we put her back in bed, she slept for a few hours, allowing me to sit down and write some thank you notes and letters to friends and family. When she woke up and began to move again, I crawled into bed with her and started to talk to her again about vacations we had taken as a family, the people who lived on our street, our pets, past Christmases, and anything else that came to mind. It was important that stimulation continue, and as Harry had said, for once my ability to talk endlessly had proven to be a gift; in fact, it was only during therapy and her naps that I did not talk to her constantly. By the end of the day, I was always tired of the sound of my own voice, but I had been told and I knew from watching the other patients at the Rehab that if recovery were to take place, it would be partly the result of all the stimulation, all the visits, all the reading, all the talking.

Later, I took Misti outside for her walk. It had snowed again, and the earth looked clean and white and pure. Suddenly, my self-pity and depression lifted, and I realized that we had not been forgotten. To have gotten this far, I was sure, God had assigned one of his very best guardian angels to Misti. I would just have to have faith and patience.

⑨

If ever there were a year when we needed the lift of spring and the Easter season, it was this one. After the small advances and many discouragements of Misti's first months at Bryn Mawr and my own loneliness, I was looking forward to seeing the entire family, who would be coming up to the Rehab for the weekend. As things turned out, though, the weekend wasn't as successful as I'd hoped. Although everyone put a brave face on the occasion, and Misti's room was soon full of Easter baskets and chocolate eggs, the family was very concerned about both Misti and me. The adults could face seeing Misti propped up in her Bryn Mawr bed or her wheelchair and even note the improvements since the last time they'd visited, but the children were very frightened and upset to see their beloved Aunt Misti thrashing around, unable to recognize them, and it took a lot of comforting and talking before they calmed down. And though everyone was very kind, it was clear that they thought that I was more than a little frazzled around the edges.

Fortunately, after the family went home things started to get better. Spring seemed to be in the air, and in response, Misti began to looked more alert. Her eyes started to lose some of the glassy coma stare, and a half smile was on her face as I dressed her and got her ready to start the week's therapies.

As always, when I took Misti down to speech therapy, I was careful to arrive early so that she would get her full forty-five minutes of therapy; unfortunately, fifteen minutes later we were still waiting. When the speech therapist finally arrived, eating cake from a staff birthday celebration, she told me that it was "just one of those things," that I would have to expect such delays from time to time. From between clenched teeth, I told her that I was sorry, but I did not expect this and, moreover, I would not accept it. If Misti was to recover, there was no time to waste. Needless to say, with this attitude, I was not likely to make points with the staff, but the old me, who was always deferential and accepting, was gone. Although I would always try to be polite, I no longer cared what they thought of me; my goal was Misti's recovery and I would not let anything stand in her way.

Later that day, after I had calmed down, I noticed a blood stain on the seat of Misti's warm-up suit. For the first time since the accident, Misti's monthly period had arrived. When I pointed this out to the nurses in Unit 700, they were very excited. They told me that this was a sure indication that the brain trauma was healing. When the brain is not working correctly, the process of menstruation does not take place. Similarly, in the time that she had been at Bryn Mawr, the diabetes that had threatened her had slowly receded. No one can be sure, but it is believed that the brain will continue to heal for about eighteen months after trauma— and however slow the process, Misti's brain did seem to be healing.

Since Terry, the occupational therapist, was pregnant and Misti was becoming more active, she began to bring in an assistant to help with Misti's therapy. With Terry and Ken working together, there were new opportunities to combine both physical and mental therapies. For instance, the physical therapists had been trying to get Misti to sit up on an exercise table with her feet dangling off it in order to improve her balance and strengthen the muscles of her torso. Of course, Misti was more likely to cooperate and less likely to be bored and become restless if she had something interesting to do or watch in the meanwhile. With two therapists available, a card game seemed like a natural for this purpose: One person could support Misti from behind while the other kept her occupied with the game.

Terry and Ken looked to me, as an expert on Misti's interests, for suggestions on a card game she might enjoy. They were surprised when I suggested poker, but the truth was, Misti had loved the game since she was a little girl. At the age of five, she had insisted that she wanted to join a poker game at a friend's picnic, and she persisted even though Harry told her it was a game for men. Amused, one of the men at the poker table let her sit on his lap and play, with Harry supplying a stake so that his friend wouldn't lose money on the proposition. Within half an hour, we heard the men at the poker table laughing and yelling: Misti had turned Harry's twenty-dollar stake into more than a hundred dollars. No one at the table could believe it, but this preschooler could actually count the cards and knew with stunning accuracy what each player had in his hands. Later, when we told Chuck and Cork about their little sister's prowess at poker, we learned that she had been winning Chuck's lunch money for weeks!

Now, years later, Misti was using those same skills again. With Ken's help she matched up the pairs and three of a kind. If Ken acted as though he were going to discard the wrong card, she became agitated. This gave everyone a certain amount of hope: Befogged though it might be, Misti's mind seemed to be working. Her brain might be bruised and the nerves battered, but there was definitely intellectual activity going on in there, and maybe there were enough undamaged parts to pick up the slack.

As I pushed Misti's wheelchair back toward her room after the therapy session, I paused at the nurse's station to have a word with Peggy. While I did, Misti's hand went to a light switch and turned off the lights in Unit 700. After turning the lights back on, we went down the hall, stopping again when Misti reached toward the water fountain. Her right hand reached out and turned the water on, while her left hand desperately tried to reach the flow of water, like Helen Keller in *The Miracle Worker*. With excitement, I turned the chair to help her reach the water; Misti let it run over her fingers, then put them into her mouth as if to suck the water from them.

By the second week of April, all the therapists noticed that Misti was more alert, more interested, more active. But progress came a bit at a time, in the usual stop-start, two-steps-forward-and-one-step-back way. One morning, after I had dressed her and opened the draperies so she could see what the weather was like, I turned back to find that Misti had stripped off her clothes and was sitting in her wheelchair, nude from the waist up, with the same devilish look she'd had as a small child when she knew she had done something wrong. Apparently, this strip-tease was Misti's latest attempt to make contact with the outside world, and she repeated the performance again and again in the next several days—and not just in her room, but in the hallway where other people were walking around. Back in her room, we chose clothing that would be hard to remove and taped garments onto Misti at the sleeves and the waist. She had clearly reached Rancho Los Amigos Level IV: She was sometimes agitated, clearly confused, and as we had just seen, had little sense of appropriate behavior. The Bryn Mawr staff and therapists were not only understanding about Misti's exhibitionist tendencies, but excited about the progress that they represented. As far as inappropriate behavior went, at a rehab facility, we saw it all: There was one young brain trauma patient, a minister's son, who spent a long time at Level V and whose vocabulary for a time consisted of nothing but a string of obscenities that would make a sailor blush, followed, incongruously enough, by the word "Coca-Cola." We would have to take this stage in stride, they said; the important thing was that Misti was making progress. And when Harry arrived later that week, he made a point of telling me that he could see just how much progress Misti was making—though he quickly got a graphic illustration of how frustrating the process could be.

Because he had been able to get away during the week, Harry was free to attend the weekly family support meeting with me. We put Misti outside her room in the chair while we went just down the hall. But before we even got to the meeting room, we heard the nurses' gentle, chiding laughter and looked back to see a half-naked girl in a wheelchair with a devilish smile on her face. Quickly, we dressed Misti again, using more tape, then secured her in her chair and pushed her out of the way of traffic before hurrying on to the support meeting. Only a few minutes later, we heard a commotion; sure that it was Misti, we bolted out the door in time to see two attendants trying to lift her from the floor from beneath her wheelchair. We had placed her too close to the wall, and she had used her right arm as a lever against it to overturn her chair. Because of the possibility of further damage to her head when she hit the floor, she had to be taken to Paoli Hospital for X-rays. Here was another problem in recovery: as her strength returned and Misti became more mobile, she also became more dangerous to herself.

The next day, as we walked toward Misti's room, we saw a new sign posted outside the door warning that no one could enter unless accompanied by a nurse. The previous evening, her biting had accelerated, and when anyone came in to check on her, she bit ferociously. The biting had been a problem for some time, but the situation was being exacerbated by her new mobility. If it continued, we were warned, we might actually have to put a muzzle on our daughter, and being told that the biting was not uncommon in recovering brain trauma patients was little consolation. In addition, Misti had started to bite her own arms, perhaps in an attempt at self-stimulation, and the nurses had to put padded mittens on her for her own protection.

The advantages of the Bryn Mawr bed became even more obvious now. If Misti were not now in this padded pen, she would have to be restrained to keep her from falling out as she thrashed and bit at the mitts like a mad animal that had been caged. Even with all the protection, she was still able to tear the bed up so much that it began to resemble a nest. Feeding Misti now became a job that took two to three people, as it was necessary to restrain her while holding the tube and injecting the liquid food.

In some ways, watching Misti's recovery from brain trauma was like watching an infant grow in awareness and competence. But whereas infants are small and helpless in their struggles, Misti was an adult in weight and power. Her age and size tempted us to try reasoning, but all talking fell on deaf ears. Each phase of recovery was different, we had learned, but this one had the potential for being the most difficult. We were grateful for the trained people at the hospital who seemed to handle the situation with ease and still maintain joy at the prospect of Misti's getting better. Without them and their experience, Harry and I might have found it impossible to cope.

When Aunt Goldie and Uncle Ora arrived with my mother and Harry's mother the following weekend, they had trouble believing that Misti was actually making progress. All they could see was Misti in the Bryn Mawr bed, thrashing and lashing out at all comers. The shock of seeing little Misti acting like a caged animal left them all with tears in their eyes. Their discouragement, on top of my own, nearly sunk me. Even Max, who was usually able to be upbeat about the possibility of Misti's recovery, seemed to be in shock at this new stage. I knew what I had been told about recovery and progression through the Rancho Los Amigos levels, but the feeling in the pit of my stomach made me want to throw up, drop to the ground, and die.

Perhaps things looked worse because I knew that shortly, I would be on my own for awhile. Worn out by the worries over Misti and the complications of his new business venture, Harry would soon be leaving for a long-planned fishing trip with an old friend in Canada. Though we were often separated by the many miles between the Rehab and Waynesboro, we spoke every day and I was secure in his support. Although I knew that Harry would only be gone for a little more than a week and that he would be calling in every other day or so, I was not looking forward to his being away. I was not sure how I could handle this difficult new phase without being able to rely on his calming strength.

For a while now, the staff at the Rehab had been talking to me about going home to Waynesboro for a visit to get some rest and recharge my batteries; they were worried, they said, that in spending so much time at the Rehab and focusing so much energy on helping Misti recover, I was endangering my own health and well-being. After a weekend like this and the prospect of even more time on my own, I was very tired and close to giving up.

The night after Harry left for home was one of those when sleep just would not come, even though there was no noise. Or maybe that was the problem—the silence, the total quiet, coupled with the knowledge that I was all alone. Every moment at the hospital was filled with therapy, laundry, reading, or talking, but once I was home the loneliness was unbearable. Though friends were terrific about writing, I was in touch with very few of them by phone. Most of them were very busy, and I guess they thought that after an exhausting day at the Rehab, the last thing I'd want to do was talk on the phone. And it was partially true: I was certainly tired each night, and I didn't feel comfortable chattering on at long distance rates when I knew how tight money was. At the same time, the town house seemed so large, each room so quiet at night. If only I knew someone here, I thought. If only there were just one person that I could talk to. To break the silence, I turned on the radio and heard Dean Martin singing "Everybody Loves Somebody." To me, the words of the song sounded more like "everybody needs somebody," so the radio proved only small comfort. After a few hours spent washing out my own clothes in the bath tub and preparing for the next day, I went to bed and, after tossing and turning for awhile, finally fell into a deep sleep.

Sometime later, I was jolted awake by the presence of a bright light that seemed to shine only on the mirror in the bedroom. The draperies were closed, so the light was not coming from outside. In fact, it seemed to be coming from nowhere at all. Next I heard footsteps coming down the hall, breaking the eerie silence, and finally, amazingly, Misti's unmistakable voice, which I had not heard in months. As I looked into the brightly lit mirror, I saw the image of her face. "Don't give up on me now—not now," she begged. Then, as quickly as the light appeared, it vanished and the dark silence was back.

In the echoing quiet of the room, I had the sudden conviction that something must be wrong with Misti, that I must get to the Rehab immediately. Quickly throwing on a pair of jeans and a sweater, I ran down the steps and out into the parking lot toward the car. As the extreme cold penetrated my feet, I realized that I was not wearing shoes, so I ran back into the house to get them. Then, I rushed back out to the parking lot and into the car, started the engine, and headed for the highway.

As I pulled into the drive at the Rehab, I looked up at the window of Misti's room, expecting to see lights. But it was dark. Quickly parking and getting out of the car, I ran to the locked door, where my cold, nervous fingers pushed an after-hours bell. When an astonished nurse answered the door a few minutes later, I explained that I must see Misti immediately; she rushed to the desk inside the door and called to Unit 700, telling them, "Mrs. Morningstar insists on coming up."

When the elevator door to the head trauma unit opened, I ran to her room as fast as my legs would carry me. The Unit 700 night nurse and I arrived at Misti's bed simultaneously; we opened the gate at its foot and peered in. Misti was breathing, but otherwise not moving. The nurse quickly used her stethoscope to listen for a heartbeat, then proceeded to take Misti's blood pressure. By this time, several puzzled nurses were in the room with us, their bewilderment turning to relief as they realized that Misti was fine, that I had just reverted to hysterical mother behavior, like a new parent who is sure that the baby has stopped breathing.

As I walked back out to the Bryn Mawr parking lot after this unnerving experience, I began to wonder if I was losing my mind. When I got back to the town house, I took a warm, relaxing bath and went back to bed, awakening what felt like only minutes later to face the trip back to the Rehab again. Had last night's events really happened? Had it all been a nightmare? Had I really been capable of driving to the Rehab and back in that state of mind? Shrugging my shoulders, I decided that it all must have been a dream.

But as I entered Unit 700, Peggy came over and asked me how I was feeling. Concern written on her face, Peggy once again urged me to consider going back to Waynesboro for a while, visiting family and friends, maybe trying to go back to work for a few days a week. I could get some rest, get myself pulled together a bit, and then return. After all, she pointed out, Misti's recovery was going so slowly that I was unlikely to miss anything significant. If I returned in a more rested, more relaxed state, she went on, I would be better able to help with Misti when she really needed me. I said I would consider the idea. I was exhausted, and I'd certainly been hearing similar suggestions from other people at the Rehab and from my own family.

Back in Misti's room, I dressed her and did her hair, chattering away as usual. Then, as I applied lipstick to her mouth and looked into her blank eyes, I recalled the words I had heard in the night, "Don't give up on me now, not now." Well, that was the answer, I thought: No matter how tired and discouraged I was, I could not forsake her now.

Partway through the day, as my tired body and foggy mind were telling me just how much sleep I'd missed the night before, Misti had a visitor from the church down the road from the Rehab: my neighbor at that first service, the lady who spoke in tongues. When she came into Misti's room, she explained that along with the gift of speaking in tongues, she also had the gift of healing. At this point, I was not about to leave any stone unturned when it came to Misti's recovery. I was not sure if this woman could help, but I was sure that she could not make matters worse. I just watched and listened quietly as she took Misti's head in her hands and said she could feel the power of God working inside her head. Then she asked if we could pray. Feeling slightly foolish, I bowed my head, and she began to pray in words not recognizable to me as any language I had ever heard.

My mind drifted off. Several years earlier, Chuck had been doing research for a paper on the subject of reincarnation. He had found a case study of a one-year-old child who seemed to be speaking a real language as he piled his toy blocks one on top of the other. This was apparently not ordinary infant babbling. Although none of the words were familiar, the boy's professor father was convinced he heard his son repeat the same words over and over and use the same inflections in each sentence. The father taped the child at play and then researched the language for months, during which time the child discontinued using the unfamiliar language and began to learn the native language of his parents. Finally, the boy's father learned that his son had been speaking an ancient Babylonian language used at the time of the building of the tower of Babel. If this could be true, who was I to discount anything that happened now?

In occupational therapy the next week, Terry put a pencil in Misti's right hand and a piece of paper in front of her on the tray of the wheelchair and asked her to write her name. In tense silence, we watched as Misti grasped the pencil and began to write. Over the course of several minutes, we saw her make one single stroke from the top of the page to about the bottom, then lift the pencil from the paper and move it over about an inch for a continuation of several scribble strokes. No letters were recognizable.

I knew that Misti had seemed much more alert lately; did she know that she was being asked to write her name? Did she even know her name? My mind drifted back to Misti as a precocious two-year-old who told me she had to learn to write her name because she wanted to show it to Dr. Kildare on TV. About thirty minutes later, she could print "MISTI," but this did not satisfy her; and two hours later she had accomplished the writing of "MORNINGSTAR" as well. I remember being so proud that I clapped. Remembering that moment now, I started to clap, though Terry seemed confused that I would clap for Misti's writing something that was not at all legible. Though it might not look like anything to most people, I was convinced that Misti's scribble was a beginning. When Harry called that evening, I told him excitedly that Misti had begun to scribble on a piece of paper. The next day in therapy Terry asked the same difficult task of Misti and again, she moved the pencil, putting forth obvious effort. Again she was rewarded with clapping and cheers. In only two days, there was great improvement in her fine-finger-control. Other therapies were harvesting similar results. In physical therapy, for instance, Karen put Misti in a swing that moved forward and backward as well as sideways. With her therapist's training, she could tell that Misti could now focus on a single object.

A day later, Misti was sitting up in her bed when I arrived in the morning. She was slumped to one side as if asleep, but there was no denying that Misti had gotten herself into a sitting position—a real accomplishment. Even though her head hung down and she was using her arm with its hard cast as a prop, she had maintained the position until I could see her. The sitting position was only the beginning. For the rest of the day, Misti rolled over and over, thrashing her legs and arms and moving broadly all over the bed. Although her left side was weaker, she clearly reveled in being able to move. By the end of the day, she had been in so many new positions that her small frail body resembled a pretzel.

When I called home that night, I had much that was positive to report to Meme Ray and Meme Semler (Misti's two grandmothers) as well as Aunt Goldie and Uncle Ora. After their shock at Misti's condition on their last visit, they all were relieved to get some good news. In fact, after many setbacks—lack of energy after intense therapies, fevers when her levels of her antiseizure medicine got too high, diarrhea when they were adjusted, the biting and agitation—things finally seemed to be running more smoothly. Misti had calmed down somewhat and had almost stopped undressing in public, the biting seemed to be passing, and she was able to stay still during her various therapies. But more was to come.

The next day, I took Misti along as usual when I went down to the cafeteria for my lunch. As we approached the dining room, the smell of food was in the air. When I looked down, Misti's right arm was twisted, her hand bent so that the fingers were almost touching the underside of her wrist. Pausing to straighten them out, I felt her fingers move in my hand. As I pulled my hand away, I realized that the motions felt deliberate, rather than random. In fact, the finger motions reminded me of the finger spelling that Misti had learned years before. Turning to face her, I said, "Misti, I do not understand what you said to me. Tell me again."

Misti had desperately wanted to learn a foreign language when she was about six years old, and we had persuaded her that American sign was a foreign language. Besides, Misti had a deaf cousin and if she learned sign, she could communicate with him. The closest finger spelling class was at Hagerstown Junior College. However, because of her age, Misti could not enroll if I did not also attend, so I had joined her there for manual communications classes. She was much faster at learning than I and soon became quite fluent. I had more difficulty, but as the years passed, we both kept up with the finger spelling, often using it as our language of choice during disagreements. If nothing else, mother-daughter arguments were quieter when conducted in sign. When Misti didn't want to "listen" anymore, she would turn her head so she could not see my signs. At that point, we usually ended up laughing, and the disagreement would come to a close.

Now, years later and under much different circumstances, I asked her to repeat what she had said and watched as her fingers formed the words, "I want French fries." Not sure if this amazing event was real or if I was having a dream because I wanted so very much for it to be happening, I repeated myself. "Sorry, Misti, my sign language is rusty; you will have to repeat that again." To my great joy she fingered, "I want French fries." Okay, I told myself, so she did it twice; it's the third time that will be the real test. Again Misti signed, "I want French fries." Dropping to my knees at the wheelchair, warm tears streaking my cheeks, I hugged her and said, "I know, I know, now we can get on with your recovery." My heart was singing. Maybe all the stimulation—the talking, the television and music, the perfume scents, and the food smells I was always trying to expose her to—was working. How extraordinary that though Misti could not yet speak, she had communicated with me. And thank God I'd been here. Who else would have noticed her finger motions and known that they meant anything? And if no one had noticed, how long might it have been before Misti gave up?

Those French fries would have to wait until Misti had recovered the ability to chew and swallow. But I couldn't wait to tell everyone what I'd just seen. Jumping to my feet, I pushed the wheelchair as fast as I could run, racing straight back to Unit 700. As soon as we arrived, I shouted, "Misti can sign! Look everyone, Misti can sign!" By this time, the nurses on the ward were accustomed to me, and remembering the last time I had been convinced that something unusual had been going on with Misti, they tried to persuade me to go home and get some rest. I would have none of this: I was not imagining the fact that my brain-injured daughter had just communicated with me for the first time in two and a half months.

Being as forceful as possible, I demanded they find someone who knew sign to verify what I knew: Misti was signing. Just as positive that I had once again gone off the deep end, they tried to convince me that I had merely witnessed the involuntary finger movements so common in brain trauma patients. A loud, nearly violent argument ensued as I insisted that they get someone who read sign to Unit 700 immediately. After I threatened to pull the Rehab down around their doubting heads, one of the nurses resignedly picked up the phone to call the Bryn Mawr administrative office. She told them that they needed someone who knew sign language in Unit 700. Although they were not enthusiastic, I was satisfied. I looked at Misti and smiled, and she smiled back—a smile that drooped on the left side because of the paralyzed muscles in her face. As I talked to her, her fingers continued to sign. I found myself wishing passionately that I had continued using the language over the past few years. Unfortunately, as the experts say, if you do not use it, you lose it, and once Misti had gone off to Mercersburg, I had fallen out of the habit of using sign language. I was paying for my negligence now: I could not read what she was trying to tell me, and the nurses did not believe that she was communicating at all.

Finally, a new face appeared in the hall, and an attractive young nurse knelt in front of Misti's wheelchair. The nurses explained to her that

"Mrs. Morningstar thinks Misti is signing, and, though this is impossible, Mrs. Morningstar will not be reasonable."

The young nurse looked into Misti's face and in a loud, clear voice said, "Hi, Mitzi, my name is Maureen and I know sign because my parents are deaf." Misti's fingers moved, and Maureen said, "Oh, excuse me." Almost in unison, the other nurses asked, "What did she say?" "Well," Maureen replied, "she said her name is not Mitzi, it's Misti."

As I tried to follow the finger-spelled conversation that ensued, I realized something else: Misti not only knew her name, but she was spelling it correctly. Chuck and Cork had chosen Misti's name, which they had heard for the first time in association with the story about the Chincoteague pony, but they had decided that rather than the standard spelling—for nothing about their baby sister was going to be standard—we should change the spelling and call her Misti.

After tucking her in bed that night, I hurried home to tell Harry the great news and share the proof that Misti was truly emerging from the coma and could now communicate with us. We had all been working so hard—Misti from within the prison of her coma, me at her bedside at the Rehab, and Harry alone in Waynesboro—all hoping and praying and looking for some sign that progress and recovery were possible, and now, with a few nonrandom movements of Misti's fingers, we had it. Harry had never been given to displays of emotion, but now, when I told him of Misti's repeated request for French fries, his voice cracked with relief and joy. In great excitement, the family passed the word from one to another. Someone on the phone chain got word to Meme Semler, and when she called the town house, she said that all things happen for a purpose, that now she realized that even something so tragic as Steven being born deaf may ultimately have had a greater purpose.

As a result of our taking a sign language class years earlier, we were now in a position to know, without question, that an essential part of Misti had survived the brain trauma and was in there, trying to get out. And after two months of terrible fear and doubt, I knew, without question, that someday—and perhaps someday soon—my daughter would come home.

Seven

Once we had established that Misti truly could communicate with me and anyone else who was able to read signed English, she immediately and spontaneously began trying to teach sign language to the nurses, therapists, and doctors who visited on Unit 700. The next day, nurses in the Rehab brought in charts showing finger spelling, and we posted them on the walls of Misti's room. Though her exhaustion at the end of each day made her rather a forlorn-looking figure, none of us was deceived: The gleam in Misti's eyes told us that she knew she had finally made a real breakthrough.

When we talked to Chuck on the phone later in the week, the conversation was less exclusively between Chuck and me and more of a three-way chat, with Misti being a more active participant, finger spelling the names of Teresa and Valera, Chuck's wife and daughter. She removed her sweatshirt only twice that day; giddy at her progress, the nurses and I could only laugh at Misti's taking her bra off over her head.

In occupational therapy, Misti continued her attempts to write her name when asked, and, although most of it was still illegible, she was clearly making both Ms and Ss and seemed to be making great progress overall, something that was confirmed when Cork and Jill brought the girls up to stay with me over the weekend. After having made so many discouraging visits, they were pleasantly surprised at the improvement in Misti's condition. For all Misti's progress, however, we were still very careful to keep Betsy and Emily at a distance, for fear that in her excitement or her frustration at not being able to communicate, Misti might bite them. And even with this precaution and evidence of progress before us, it was clear that four-year-old Emily was still afraid of Misti. The wheelchair and Misti's somewhat wild appearance—her head was still held up by a halo on the wheelchair—were very unfamiliar to both of the little girls, who had trouble reconciling this figure with the Aunt Misti they remembered.

Misti spent one whole day of the weekend attempting to teach Max and his parents sign language; Max was able to pick up enough to get the gist of Misti's conversation and acted as interpreter for his parents. Harry was also able to make the trip up that weekend and was thrilled to see Misti begin to communicate. Unfortunately, in his state of exhaustion, learning sign language proved to be too much for him; try

78

as he might, he always had to have someone else present as a translator.

As the weeks passed, Misti continued to sign and, perhaps because she was so much less frustrated in her attempts to communicate, largely stopped biting. But in the torturous way of recovery from brain trauma, one troubling behavior soon replaced another, and now she began to pinch people—and quite painfully—when she wanted their attention or felt she wasn't getting through quickly enough.

One of the first things that Misti communicated was that she was tired of wearing diapers and was ready to learn to use the bathroom by herself again. Surprisingly, we had to fight to get this taken care of. Typically, patients who've suffered strokes, spinal cord injury, and brain trauma do not make great progress with such matters. When they are released from the rehab facility to the community, most of them are still in adult-care diapers and often do not recover conventional bowel and bladder function. And, I was told, toilet retraining would be difficult now because Misti's bladder would have shrunk. Still, we persisted: This was what Misti actively wanted, and we would go along, with me in charge of the process. We explained all this to Misti, and when I talked with her about the plan, I found myself remembering a conversation we'd had when she was sixteen months old and informed me that she wanted to stop wearing diapers and start wearing "big girl pants." Not long after, we put away the diapers and dressed Misti in training under-pants, and in a remarkably short time, she was toilet trained. My hope now was that accomplishing this new task would be as easy—and it was. Despite the staff's concern, Misti was on a regular schedule and out of diapers within three weeks.

At the same time, there was a new challenge for Misti: Now that we knew she could indeed hear and understand conversation and reply, we had to persuade her to move beyond sign language toward vocal com-munication. When I got to the Rehab on Monday morning, Peggy was lying in the Bryn Mawr bed with Misti, and I could hear her saying, "Come on Misti, like your mother says, you're a Morningstar, you can do it." Over and over, Peggy encouraged Misti to blow, to move her tongue, and try to get out a sound.

Karen, the speech therapist, explained that the voluntary muscles of the mouth, throat, and tongue had to be retrained if Misti was to be able to communicate in the usual way again. There were three basic skills Misti needed to master before she could talk again. First, she would need to be able to blow with some force; second, she would need to be able to stick out her tongue; and third, she would need to be able to push each cheek out with her tongue.

When Harry arrived for a short stay the following weekend, he spent hours diligently trying to get Misti to blow. A master of motivation, he remembered that Misti had become totally infatuated with a blue stuffed dog in the Bryn Mawr gift shop. Now he told her that she would get the dog when she could blow to his satisfaction. Every day, he held a hand in front of Misti's mouth and seemed crestfallen when he could not feel any air coming out of her mouth. He'd hold Misti's hand up to his mouth while he blew and asked her if she could feel it, then reverse the process, holding her hand in front of her mouth and telling her again to blow. This went on hour after hour, day after day, for several weeks, with me taking over when Harry went back to Waynesboro.

Karen also suggested that it was time to try to get Misti to swallow, since as soon as she was able to swallow, she would be able to start to learn to eat again. And perhaps in the near future the feeding tube in her abdomen could be removed. We did talk to Misti about the swallow therapy, so she would know what to expect, but we didn't discuss the longer range goal of eating. I felt that to do so would be cruel; at this point, she couldn't do it, so why raise her hopes until we were closer to the goal and had a better sense of what was really possible?

We made the first try at swallow therapy using finely ground ice, putting small pieces into Misti's mouth. It was clear that she enjoyed the feeling, but she couldn't seem to get the hang of swallowing and the ice melted, running out of her mouth and over her clothes. The next attempt was made by another therapist, a swallow expert, who brought in raspberry ice and a small spoon, again putting a small amount of the flavored ice in Misti's mouth. Again, it was plain that she enjoyed the taste and feeling, like a small child relishing a new experience. She tried very hard to swallow, so the raspberry ice would not melt and run out of her mouth. After an hour of great effort, she was tired, but when the therapist told her what a good job she had done, Misti smiled, using her right hand to push the left side of her face up with her fingers.

Just as Misti had begun to finger spell "bed" and "sleep," Harry walked into the room, his eyes gleaming with the excitement of a having made a great discovery. He had gone into town and bought a new toy for Misti—not the blue dog, but a bottle of bubbles. He dipped the wand into the soapy liquid and began to blow bubbles, then invited her to blow bubbles, too. She tried and tried, then Harry blew some more bubbles. Finally, exhausted, she begged to go to sleep and was sound asleep within minutes. Since Misti's attempts to communicate had became clearer, hopes for greater recovery and expectations of her had risen sharply, with therapy sessions becoming more intense. These days she seemed to actively welcome the weekends, when the regularly scheduled therapies stopped and she could get more rest. At this point, her erratic night sleep patterns had normalized, and she was sleeping through the night and taking two naps during the day, sometimes for as long as two or three hours at a time.

Patiently, Harry sat at Misti's bedside and waited for her to awaken and then move back into the wheelchair. When she did, the two again went through the exercise of blowing bubbles. The therapists were so pleased with Harry's idea that they said they would use it with other patients. It seemed amazing that something so simple could become such a valuable tool.

Later, we put Misti back in bed, relaxed a bit, and caught up on reading some of the many cards and notes that friends had sent to Misti. Suddenly, Misti turned over, and a groaning sound rolled through her diaphragm and exploded in a belch from her mouth—the first sound to come from her since the accident and a sure sign that we were on the right track with the various therapies aimed at helping Misti get ready to talk once again.

We all had a very full week. Day after day, we helped Misti practice sticking out her tongue by sticking out our tongues. What a sight: a mature building developer, a seasoned interior designer, and a seventeen-year-old recovering from brain trauma, cheering each other on as we all tried sticking out our tongues as far as possible! The only thing funnier was seeing the three of us trying to touch our noses and chins with our tongues. But silly-looking or not, the fact remained: Once the tongue is maneuverable, the forming of words can become a reality.

Further progress was temporarily derailed when Misti and all the other patients on the unit came down with the flu. But after a few days, everything got back to normal. Blowing therapy resumed, becoming a major task. When one day Misti blew hard enough and the liquid stretched on the wand and yielded the first little round bubble, the beauty of the light reflecting from the iridescent miracle brought cheers that could be heard over the entire unit. With great anticipation, Misti then turned to Harry, finger spelling "blue dog." Tender perfectionist that he is, Harry told her that she could not yet have the dog, that she had produced only one bubble, that we needed to see more. And with that they returned to the task of transforming the soapy liquid into beautiful air-filled globes.

Back at the town house that night, Harry and I discussed the miracle of watching someone come back to life. For years, we had had the pain of watching the brain deteriorate as my father slipped into the dark semideath of Alzheimer's; now the process was being reversed as we watched Misti emerge from the semideath of coma.

After all the effort he had put into teaching Misti to blow, Harry had to leave the next day to go back to Waynesboro. I often thought about him making that long and quiet trip back home each weekend—exhausted, wishing, hoping, praying, and worrying. I knew that he would have preferred to stay at Bryn Mawr with me and continue watching the miracle take place, but he was responsible for earning the money to pay for this process. Rehabs are not inexpensive, and unfortunately, the better the institution, the more it costs. We had jointly decided that Misti's recovery would require the best, and so we had chosen Bryn Mawr. We had been getting help from Pennsylvania's CAT insurance fund. This fund provided coverage through driver's license fees and was used to help the victims of catastrophic accidents deal with bills between $100,000 and $1 million, where our private catastrophic coverage would kick in, but we were starting to hear rumblings that the fund was running very low. Since I was tending to Misti, our family was without my income, and at the same time we had the expenses of an extra apartment plus utilities, not to mention my meals and the cost of daily transportation. This meant that Harry's income was essential to keeping Misti's recovery on track.

Only minutes after Harry reluctantly departed, the physical therapist came into Misti's room with a strange-looking apparatus. It looked like a large walker with a padded top shaped like a horseshoe. Having had no previous experience with rehabilitation, I had not even known such things existed, and I sent out a prayer of thanks to the ingenious engineers and therapists who had worked together to come up with such unlikely-looking but useful devices. I now watched the therapists lift Misti's frail body onto this thing, draping her arms over the padded top and letting her legs, weighed down by the two heavy white casts, dangle to the floor. Karen sat down on a small four-legged stool with wheels behind Misti, holding her firmly at the hips. Karen's assistant, facing Misti, moved slowly backward while holding Misti's arms over the soft top. Maneuvering carefully thus, the two proceeded to push one of Misti's cast-clad legs in front of the other.

Each day brought more surprises and more joy, but with each bit of progress came more work. With plenty of encouragement from everyone, Misti continued to work diligently, and we duly recorded each new effort on videotape. When the rehab staff questioned me about the filming, I explained that Misti would surely want to see them when she had recovered and would want to know exactly what happened. My answer was not what the experts wanted to hear, and in their own ways all of the doctors, nurses, and social workers tried to prepare me for what they considered the necessary and inevitable jolt of reality. Quietly, patiently, they explained that even though she was no longer in much physical danger of dying, Misti would not make a truly substantial recovery from the brain trauma. The sooner I accepted the fact, the better for everyone. I was told in gentle but firm terms that the high hopes and expectations I had for her were very unrealistic. Though Misti was now able to communicate, and though she might yet learn to eat on her own again, she would never be able to propel her own wheelchair or go to college; she might never even be able to care for her own personal needs. My argument that she was improving markedly brought further kind explanations that, though this might be true, time was passing without enough concrete results to suggest real recovery.

Considering their words as I bathed Misti that night, I was newly and painfully aware of the helplessness of her limbs. Later, back in my room at the townhouse, depression dropped down on me. The words from the Bryn Mawr staff earlier in the day echoed silently through the lonely, empty room: "Time is passing by." Compounding my worries for Misti were my concerns for Harry, who was working very hard to pay for the rehabilitation services not covered by our insurance or the CAT fund. So far Harry's work was keeping our heads above water, but he was having to draw on our hard-earned retirement savings to pay for such essentials as rent and long distance service at Chesterbrook. And who knew how much longer this would take? Mightn't the experts be right and Misti not recover much more?

The next day was full of the painful paradox of rehabilitative therapy. Speech therapy ground on without yielding audible results, but when asked by the therapist what was in the sky, Misti finger spelled "stars," "sun," "moon," "planets," "constellations," and "clouds." At noon, when apple sauce and ice cream were brought in for a joint attempt at lunch and swallow therapy, I watched in silence as small amounts of the food were put to Misti's lips and she tried with great effort to contain the semiliquids in her mouth and prevent them from running out onto her bibbed chest. For all my hopes and optimism, I was forced to recognize that the Bryn Mawr staff might be right about Misti's ultimate inability to take care of herself.

I was nearly undone later that night when I discovered that the electricity was out in the entire Chesterbrook development, which meant that I couldn't even take the long hot bath that was one of my few relaxing pleasures. I fell asleep remembering what my friend Dixie always said: "God will not give you more than you can bear." With this in mind, I offered up my own sardonic prayer: "God, you'd better stop soon, because I have had just about enough."

I did not need an alarm to wake up the next morning. But on the ride to the Rehab, I wondered if I would ever get enough sleep again. I was so tired that I felt I could go to sleep and not wake up, ever. But then who would help Misti?

Realizing that you sometimes must have clouds to see the silver lining, I walked into the Rehab to find Misti sitting up in her chair. She had already been fed breakfast. Her bib was caked with pulverized food; there was more on the nurse, the chair, and the tray. However messy the room, though, Misti had been able to take in enough food to make it clear that she could indeed swallow if an attendant was able to persevere. That meant that perhaps not too long into the future, we might be able to get rid of the feeding tube.

After the necessary major clean up, we headed for therapy. When Marilyn, her cognitive retraining therapist, selected a photo from a box into which we'd put pictures of friends and family members over the last several months, Misti spelled the name of the person in the photo. Unfortunately, this did not prove that she remembered the person in question because she had been shown the photos often over the months and told the identities of those pictured.

When Marilyn asked if there was anything special she would like to do today, Misti finger spelled "mirror." A hand-held mirror was produced and held in front of her. Misti wanted to see her face. She tried to get as close as possible to the mirror, with her glasses tapping against its surface. After staring at herself for a few minutes, a smile of what seemed to be relief crossed her face. Perhaps this was because we had never explained to her exactly how much damage had been done to her from the accident, preferring to focus on the positive. Perhaps this was because she had not really been able to take in what we did tell her. Or perhaps she had been worried about something else altogether. After months at Bryn Mawr, I knew that we could only wonder what was going on in her mind and what questions she would ask if she could.

While Misti was resting later that day, the phone rang. When I answered it, it was easy to recognize the cheerful voice of Rani Carnicello, Misti's best friend since the age of four. Rani is a happy conversationalist, able to bubble and carry on a conversation with only occasional response from the listener, and I knew Misti would enjoy hearing from her. I told Misti that it was Rani and that she wanted to speak to her. As I held the phone to her ear, I recognized her excitement at listening to someone she loved so much—and her frustration at having to expend such a great effort to make words. Ultimately, she tried so hard with so little result that she became highly irritable and started to bite, pushing the phone away. Then, quite suddenly, I felt an immense blow to my crotch. As pain ripped through my body and I dropped to the floor, I realized that Misti was now able to lift her right leg and move the heavy cast with great force. It was hard to tell which was worse—the emotional pain and shock or the physical pain. Knowing that she did not know what she was doing and that she would not even remember the incident in another minute did not help. I'd witnessed the biting and the pinching, but this was the first time one of her coming-out-of-coma behaviors had Misti's full force behind it, and it was devastating.

After the phone call, Rani talked with her mother and they decided to drive up to see Misti in person the next day. When they arrived at Bryn Mawr, an excited Misti wanted to go to the cafeteria with them. Bonnie and Rani thought it best if I were to go along; I had the feeling they were leery of taking her without me as backup. At the cafeteria, Bonnie and I sat at one table and allowed Misti and Rani to have some privacy. After the previous day's experience, I was worried that Misti would bite or pinch Rani when she leaned in close and whispered in her ear. I watched closely for any sign that she might act up again, then noticed with relief that Misti's responses to Rani were in sign. And not just ordinary sign. As we watched the girls, Bonnie realized that Misti was using Pig Latin in sign language. Her use of the language she and Rani had sometimes spoken as children definitely proved that her brain was recovering function.

Before Bonnie and Rani left for the evening, they helped give Misti her shower, and the sounds emanating from the shower room almost made everyone forget the seriousness of our lives now. Good laughter, silly giggles, and white soap bubbles filled the room, and it was possible to believe that life once again would be good.

☺

As spring moved toward summer, intense therapy of every kind continued, and the VCR camera kept rolling. One memorable day, Karen, the physiotherapist, draped Misti's body face down over a thirty-six-inch cylinder of red plastic. Then, with Karen helping from behind, and her assistant from the front, Misti rolled back and forth over the plastic cylinder. With each roll Karen said, "I hear air coming out. Try to form a word and say something as the air comes out." I knew that the therapists knew their jobs, but after months without hearing Misti's voice, I had no real sense of expectation. Then I watched Misti lift her head up and look directly at me. To my shocked amazement, the glorious words "Hi, Mom" belched from her mouth.

If I live to be a hundred, I know I will never appreciate or enjoy anything as much as that single second when Misti said her first words in her new life. The joy of earlier occasions of Misti's life—when I learned that a baby girl was available for the Morningstar family, when she was put in my arms for the first time, when I watched her take her first trembling steps—was far exceeded by the ecstasy I felt as I took in those two simple but wonderful words. Tears fell from my eyes and blurred my vision.

Misti was making progress on all fronts now. If anyone had ever deserved to earn a prize, Misti now did for persevering through the tedium of relearning to blow. After weeks of increasingly effective practice, we all agreed that her efforts had earned her the blue dog. When Harry brought the stuffed animal in, Misti finger-spelled a request for his name. Harry told her that the toy's tag read "Fuffer," but Misti shook her head in disagreement and insistently spelled out "Blow." We all laughed at the name that could not have been more appropriate.

Back in Chesterbrook that night, Harry and I discussed the gift we'd been given when Misti had learned sign language all those years ago. We wondered aloud how many other brain injured patients were trying just as hard as Misti to emerge from coma, but were stymied because they had no way of showing or telling anyone that they could recover further. If I had not been there to recognized Misti's so-called involuntary finger movements as communication, how long would it have been before she had given up and gone blank in frustration?

At that moment, it truly came home to us how important it is for a recovering brain trauma patient to have a loved one close by at all times. While trained rehabilitation workers do work miracles, they often do not recognize the little signs that a mother, father, or mate can identify as a patient's possible effort to communicate. Although it wasn't easy and we were certainly feeling the strain—emotional, physical, and financial—Harry and I were very grateful to have been in a position to be able to rearrange our jobs and other family obligations in order to devote the time to Misti's recovery. In many families, unfortunately, it is impossible for either a parent or a spouse to devote themselves full-time to helping with recovery.

I was exquisitely thankful for each day I was able spend with her, as was Harry. And yet here we faced another dilemma: We all recognized that when Harry was able to be at the Rehab with us, everything seemed to go much better. Misti made more progress, and Harry and I were able to lean on each other when the frustrations and upsets proved overwhelming. However, Harry simply could not stay with us all the time. Someone had to work to fill the chasm between what the insurance covered and what Misti needed—especially now that it looked as though the CAT fund was about to run dry. We both knew and accepted this, but it was very, very hard on the entire family.

※

With the help of all kinds of exercises, Misti's verbal attempts to communicate were slowly improving, though at this point she didn't have much wind power, and the sounds she could make were still very faint. And because Misti's left side was still partially paralyzed, interfering with the coordination of the muscles of her mouth and throat, her speech tended to be slurred in addition to faint. This meant that I was forced even deeper into the role of Misti's interpreter.

On the physical therapy front, exercises of all sorts continued. One especially interesting exercise involved draping Misti's body over a large orange ball, which forced Misti to use her neck muscles reflexively to hold up her head. Another day she was introduced to a grocery shopping cart, which allowed her to practice walking and balance. It was still a three-person operation: With painstaking efforts, Karen, her assistant, and Misti all fought to keep Misti's body in an erect position behind the cart. As part of her routine, Misti was allowed to placed the various stuffed toys she'd accumulated in the cart, which she slowly maneuvered through the unit. An advantage of this therapy was that Misti was able to recover some of her elementary social skills. She loved to sneak up on her favorite nurse, Peggy, and startle her by calling her name as loud as possible. Every time, Peggy jumped as though she had been frightened by the loud scream, then turned to Misti with a hug and a laugh.

On the occupational therapy front, the job was harder, the progress less easy to discern. Misti might forget something that had just happened—especially if it was connected to some kind of emotion, such as frustration—but focus intently on things like getting the blue dog. We couldn't even know how much she remembered from the distant past. Because we had talked to her about everything, it was quite possible that the memories she had were ones that we'd planted.

Misti was still tiring very easily from the hard work of therapy and significant levels of antiseizure medicine, and she often begged to stay in bed, or go back to bed, or to go to bed early. Each day we tried to keep her up a few minutes longer, attempting to increase her stamina. To that end, we put a watch on her left arm, hoping that its presence there would encourage her to strengthen those weaker muscles by using them to bring the watch to her face to see the time. One day, after Linda told her that she must wait until 4:00 before she could take her nap, Misti worked diligently to lift her left arm up, and then, summoning all her energy and using every fine motor skill she had recovered, she changed the position of the hands on the watch and tried to persuade Linda that it was already 4:00. This kind of problem solving reminded me of a small child trying to make sense of the universe and the commands and demands of adults.

Similarly, even as the staff introduced Misti to the call buzzer she could use to summon a nurse, we all realized they might be creating a monster. Quite predictably, as soon as Misti figured out how to use the buzzer, she began to overuse it. At this stage of her rehabilitation, she was like a child who had learned a new skill or gotten a new toy. Or perhaps it was merely that after months of frustrating passivity, she was reveling in her new sense of autonomy and ability to communicate her desires.

Even though every new advance pointed to recovery, there were inevitably disquieting times when we all realized that Misti's brain was just not functioning properly, and perhaps it would not recover any further. She sometimes seemed not to recognize basic facts about her life at present, such as her inability to get around under her own steam. Then there were the other frustrations that go with recovery from coma, such as when Misti began sticking her tongue out when thwarted. Ironically, one of the things we'd worked hardest to help Misti regain—the ability to stick out her tongue—had become one of the things we now had to teach her not to do.

One of the elements of physical therapy for Misti involved balancing on a swing attached to the ceiling by four ropes and equipped with a safety back. One day when Misti was on the swing, the therapist paid especially close attention to Misti's eyes as she was pushed back and forth and then from side to side. As she watched Misti attempt to focus, she could tell there were some problems with Misti's vision. She pointed out what we could see when we looked more closely: Misti's eyes were out of alignment. One eye turned inward and its focal point was higher than the other. From the time Misti had been batting at the balloons, we'd known she was not seeing as well as she should, and this was professional confirmation. Further, this vision problem might be part of the reason for Misti's slow progress with the physical therapy and fine-motor-skill development; even if Misti's injured brain were recovering, she would obviously have problems if she wasn't seeing properly.

Back in her room that afternoon, we were greeted by Rani and another of Misti's friends, Heather. I left the three girls alone together in Misti's room so they could have some privacy. As I went out into the hall, the giggles and laughter I could hear reminded me of happier times in the past, when I'd pass Misti's closed bedroom door and hear music playing and the three girls talking and giggling late into the night. When they finally emerged from the room, with Heather and Rani pushing Misti's chair out to the hall, we stopped to admire the new hairstyle they had created for her. Misti was all smiles that afternoon, but when the time came for the girls to leave, she started to laugh—not a natural, spontaneous, hearty laugh, but one that was strange, uncanny, like the sound of the fat lady in a carnival or a laugh track on a bad sitcom. Whatever it was, it worried me.

At the next team meeting, Marilyn, the cognitive therapist, announced her plans to reintroduce Misti to a computer. On it, they would play word, math, and video games, match shapes, and use the keyboard to create cards, letters, and drawings, all the while trying to retrain the undamaged portions of Misti's brain, build up her fine-finger-motion skills, and strengthen her memory. Only a year before the computer had become Misti's best buddy when it was time for homework, so we hoped she would accept this readily.

The team also announced that a neuro-ophthalmologist would visit Misti and try to nail down the problem with her eyes, and Misti would continue walking behind the grocery cart as a balance exercise. Best of all came the news that the heavy, bulky casts could finally be removed from Misti's legs and exercises could start to stretch her tendons without them. This was terrific news because Misti couldn't easily control the casts, which meant that much of her skin was covered with bruises. And once the casts were off, she could make faster progress in physical therapy because their weight impeded her movements a lot.

That weekend, Brenda and Anthony brought Max up to the Rehab, and with the help of Max, who had assumed the job of sign interpreter for his parents, Misti informed us that she had a surprise. Her eyes sparkled brightly as she told her audience that she was now eating so well that her feeding tube would be removed on Monday. When I asked the nurses on the unit why this had not been discussed in group meeting, they looked startled and fumbled through Misti's chart for any mention of the feeding tube. There was no such notation. One thing was now clear, however: Misti had learned to lie.

No one had prepared me for the fact that Misti would learn to lie, but one of the nurses told me that this unsettling development was actually a further sign of recovery. Although most patients on the unit would say whatever might cross their minds, they didn't have sufficient reasoning ability to formulate lies. And whereas I'd have scolded the child Misti for being mischievous in making up a story, I couldn't scold her for lying now. Instead, when she lied, we just laughed at the situation and told her that of course we knew she was making things up.

Another aspect of Misti's recovery came into play a few days later, when my mother made a visit. She was alarmed to see Misti's face go into contortions and immediately wanted to know what hurt. In response Misti finger spelled, "I'm winking at Meme." I was at once reminded of Misti as a little kid, experimenting with her world and in the process, learning to tease, learning to make a joke, to snap her fingers, or whistle, or wink.

⑨

Four to five weeks after she began swallow therapy, Misti had graduated to eating enough baby food to keep her nourished. Though therapy to encourage Misti to eat solid food would continue, the team decided that her feeding tube could finally be removed. After a trip to Paoli Hospital, the only remaining sign of Misti's detour into artificial nourishment was a Band-Aid on her stomach to mark the spot where the tube had protruded for so long.

On April first, Misti decided to play a joke on the nurses and stay in bed for the day, but they didn't fall for it and soon had her out of bed and working hard. That first Friday of the month was also time for the larger group meeting. The doctor who chaired the meeting began by announcing that unfortunately, the Morningstars' insurance had now run out and Misti could no longer stay at Bryn Mawr. Everyone was terribly disappointed and rushed to express regret: Misti had made such great strides here, far surpassing other patients; she might regress without the constant therapies here; wasn't there some way she could stay? The doctor then said, "April Fool's! Now let's continue with the meeting." Though I could have done without the heart-stopping joke (now that the CAT fund had gone bankrupt, we were very concerned about money and the cost of the Rehab) I was actually heartened by this meeting. I knew the joke hadn't been directed at me, and I also knew that, despite their instinctive, protective caution, the entire staff at the Rehab was pulling for Misti and would have been crushed if she had had to leave before they had done all they could for her.

Later in the day, the familiar brown Mercersburg van pulled up with Mr. Needham and his load of students, ready for a visit and carrying mail from school. Included were Misti's college acceptance letters and information about graduation and class standing at Mercersburg. As Mr. Needham read the words "Honors for Misti Morningstar," she started to laugh—again, not a laugh that seemed normal, but that same animal-like laugh I'd heard when Rani and Heather were visiting. The kids who were visiting were visibly alarmed and confused by this turn of events. No matter how many times they were told that recovery from brain trauma was unpredictable and confusing, it was hard for them to reconcile these facts with the behavior of their classmate here at the Rehab, and it was always disconcerting for them.

As the talk turned to graduation, Mr. Needham assured Misti that she would graduate with her class, and she replied that she would be there. As they all prepared to leave, she signed that the next time they came to visit, she would leave with them and they would all stop at Burger King. It was hard to watch the kids' reactions as they said good-bye to Misti. I knew she was recovering, but she had no real idea of the extent of her mental or physical deficits, and to many of the kids, she looked as though she had scarcely recovered at all.

Mr. Needham's visit to Bryn Mawr brought up a new challenge: We had to get Dr. Audieh to agree that Misti could go to the Mercersburg graduation. Dr. Audieh was hesitant to approve the trip because there was no way to know whether or how much more Misti would recover, and she was afraid to jeopardize possible future progress by allowing her to get into a situation where she would be forced to confront her deficits before she could cope. At the next team meeting, we discussed trying to take Misti out of the Rehab for a few hours at a time—in the car, perhaps to a restaurant—with the goal of trying to reintroduce her to the outside world gradually, before making any future plans for a big outing like graduation.

When I asked Dr. Audieh's about the strange laughter that had been emanating from Misti at inappropriate times, she told me that in some brain trauma patients, the emotional processing center gets damaged and emotions can get mixed up. After I told her of the circumstances surrounding Misti's episodes of canned laughter, she told me that in Misti's brain, the responses for crying and laughing may have gotten turned around. Because each case of brain trauma is so different, she couldn't offer any real prognosis that this situation might improve at some point. As with so much of recovery from brain trauma, today's behavior provides clues only about tomorrow's actions, not about long-term prospects for betterment of the patient's condition. We would all have to wait and see.

Eight

In preparation for our first trip outside the institution, it was time to get Misti out of the large, rather clumsy wheelchair she'd been using and into something more streamlined and easier to transport. She no longer needed all of the attachments on the big wheelchair. In physical therapy, they'd been working hard at getting her to hold her head up without the help of the halo, and she was succeeding in keeping it erect more of the time now.

After several weeks away, Harry returned to Bryn Mawr for a visit and heard, for the first time, of the great plans Misti had been making-her hopes of attending the Mercersburg graduation, of going out with friends for pizza—all presented with Misti's characteristic determination to accomplish everything the very next day. While we were heartened to see this return of the old Misti, we were also much aware that she wasn't thinking very practically. Though she could not walk or even talk understandably, Misti was convinced that she was just about well. There was a huge gap between her understanding of her situation and her desire to return to the life she had known. She was not especially agitating to leave the Rehab; she just felt she was ready to go back to participating in life.

Now back on regular, though still pulverized, food, Misti was determined to feed herself. She was actually succeeding in getting a good amount of the food in her mouth and then down to her stomach. Her biggest problem was with drinking liquids. Even a few drops of water could cause her to choke, sending liquid into her lungs instead of down her esophagus to her stomach. One morning we had to get X-rays of her lungs taken to see if any of the liquids or baby food had gone into them, which could lead to pneumonia, among other problems. The wonderful reply was negative; in this case, everything seemed to be working efficiently.

After a few weeks, a new blue wheelchair arrived, greeted by cheers from us. Despite the fact that the CAT fund had balked at spending an extra fifteen dollars to get a wheelchair in red, which Misti really would have preferred, there was nevertheless a sparkle in her eyes, as she signed, "I always wanted my own wheels." The new chair had no supports; her task now was to learn to keep her arms on the armrests and concentrate on holding up her head unassisted. Without a tray, she had to learn to keep her hands on her lap, or they would just dangle at her sides. She was delighted that the chair could fold up. That meant it could be put it in the trunk of the car and we could leave the grounds of the Rehab for outings.

Of course, once the chair arrived, Misti was determined that the outing must be immediate—that very day. However, she would need a lot of practice with maneuvering the new chair and sitting comfortably and controllably in it. Fortunately, a trip to the car to see that the wheelchair would in fact fit into the trunk plus a lesson on transferring her from the chair to the car seat was enough to satisfy the day's ambitions.

Back in the head trauma unit, Misti agreed to let us set up the VCR and view some of the videotapes we had been making since early March. Until this time, she had refused to watch them, but today, the timing of the tape seemed perfect. However, after watching just five minutes of the tape, she became restless and reacted violently to the film, wanting to have nothing more to do with it.

Later, the eye doctor arrived to examine Misti for new glasses, which he said would arrive in about ten days. He was confident that the new lenses, which were designed to correct some of the misalignment she'd suffered in the accident, could help her see better. He hoped they would enable her to handle therapies in a more positive and productive way. Another part of the plan was for Misti to start using patches over one eye at a time to build up strength in her eye muscles and give her some relief from the misaligned vision.

My early, fearfully modest dreams and hopes were becoming a reality. Once she had learned to balance, Misti was able to propel the new light weight wheelchair with her right foot, and although she could not yet make it go in a straight line—the paralysis on her left side was still apparent—God be praised, she could move her chair about two feet by herself! In just three short months at Bryn Mawr, Misti had accomplished an enormous amount, so much more than the doctors ever thought possible.

After getting her ready for bed that night, I sat with her for a long while and told her how proud I was of her and all that she was able to do. I offered reassurance that she might be able to go back to Mercersburg Academy and graduate, go on to college, have a career, marry, and be happy. After all, since she had come this far, nothing should stop her now! There was no one to stop me offering my hopes for her, no one standing there whispering that her progress was incremental at best.

Soon after the new wheelchair arrived, Misti was scheduled to attend craft therapy for the first time. Everyone in the craft class was handicapped, and many were in worse shape than Misti, but there were some who could walk using canes or walkers. These were people who had once held responsible positions in their communities, mothers or fathers who provided for families, young people with promising futures. One member of the class was a police officer who had been rammed head-on in the patrol car while in pursuit of a drug gang. As a result, he was unable to talk and largely unable to think. I could only wonder how the world would have been changed if these people had not been brutally cut off from more normal life so soon.

At Bryn Mawr and at home in Waynesboro, excitement continued to run high as Misti's recovery sped on. Though busy with their own lives, everyone in the family was happy to hear that Misti was doing better and hopeful that we would soon be able to return to Waynesboro. Of course, their notion of returning to "real life" was not based on seeing Misti's rehabilitation day by day, and I wasn't sure what context they had for gauging the small, hard-won daily victories that we were reporting. Meanwhile, Misti was becoming more independent, learning to get from her wheelchair to bed without assistance. That she could sit up in bed alone and was able to talk more each day gave me confidence that one day she would be able to do all the things she wanted to. One proud day, she was transferred from the pen-type Bryn Mawr bed that had served her so well to a standard hospital bed.

In therapy she was learning to get around in a kitchen that had been set up for wheelchair-bound people, and as a part of occupational therapy, she learned to make chocolate chip cookies. Most exciting of all, in physical therapy, she had learned how to transfer herself from the wheelchair to a car seat. The Rehab continued to test her blood to check Tegretol levels, and new casts were made to help stretch the muscles that had tightened from lack of use, but progress was definitely taking place.

The next step for Misti was to enter the Protected Unit, where patients had the freedom to move around by themselves with supervision only when they needed it. This unit was housed behind locked doors with a code access restricted for nurses. It was both amusing and somewhat sad to watch the patients try to figure ways to get through the locked doors, many of them explaining that they had to get out to go home.

One young man explained to me that he had to leave the unit because his family was waiting for him to come home to celebrate his daughter's first birthday. When I refused to help him, he got angry and started to curse and scream at me. A nurse hurried to restrain him, explaining that he was always trying to talk people into letting him out to get to his daughter. In reality, his daughter was now in grade school and came to see him with her mother about once a month. Sadly, when they came to visit, he never recognized them. His last solid memory was of driving home from work to celebrate the little girl's first birthday. A drunk driver ran a red light and the rest was history—just another statistic in the traffic court, but one that left a family shattered.

Visitors for Misti still came from the Academy, as well as friends and relatives from Waynesboro. All were pleased to see her improvement, but it was becoming obvious that they did not expect Misti to return to school or graduate. Still, the staff at the Rehab seemed to be coming around somewhat and no longer necessarily shared this gloomy view. They seemed prepared to help Misti go as far as possible, and as she mastered more elements of rehabilitative therapy, they helped formulate new goals for her.

The woman from the local church who spoke in tongues continued to make her weekly visits to Misti, offering prayers in her unusual language and trying her healing powers. While initially Misti had seemed unaware of the woman, now she seemed to be taking her in—and clearly was not terrifically comfortable. "Who is this person?" her sidewise looks to me asked. Still, the woman obviously meant well; Misti was always polite and I was always glad to have another person's prayers made on Misti's behalf.

One day, a new and rather unbelievable form of new therapy was suggested for Misti: horseback riding. My daughter, who was still partially paralyzed from the head trauma, would soon be riding a horse? The notion that this form of recreational therapy could be helpful to someone in Misti's position seemed amazing to me until one of the therapists explained that riding a horse bareback causes the muscles in the pelvis to work the same way that they do when one is walking. I was assured that the horses in question had been specially trained to do their job, and it was clear that this was true. The horses were very gentle, and Misti, secured on hers with a belt around her waist with special handles on each side, could not have been safer. Each handle was held by a therapist, who walked beside the horse, while another member of the team led the large and docile animal around a track. Even in the riding stable, there were special ramps to accommodate the wheelchairs and help lift the patient from the chair onto the back of the horse. Misti especially enjoyed this therapy and not least because we had to get out of Bryn Mawr and into the car for the five-minute ride down the road to the farm.

Now that Misti had a portable wheelchair and had learned to help with transfers, it was time to plan a real outing for her. The nurses and therapists were in on the planning, and we all worked hard to make the dream a reality. Midweek, two friends from Harrisburg and their son volunteered to come to the Rehab, and together we took Misti out for her great adventure: a trip to the local Crab Shanty for dinner. She was concerned that we would all be embarrassed by her appearance and lack of coordination, but we all assured her that that was not the case. Since Misti was eating some solid foods by this time, she could order mashed potatoes and other foods that could be easily cut up, and we could help her eat.

In planning for the outing, we'd tried to anticipate anything that could present a problem and deal with it in advance so that we could all have a good time. However, once we arrived at the restaurant, we realized that we'd missed a crucial step: We hadn't considered the problem of getting Misti into the restaurant, which had four steps to the door. Thankfully, with two strong men to carrying the wheelchair, we managed to make it to our table without much trouble. Once we began ordering, another problem arose when the waitress had difficulty understanding Misti when she tried to place her order. She was not very polite about it: "I don't understand her at all. Can't she talk plainer?" We would simply refuse to let this ignorant person upset us, I explained to Misti in front of the waitress, mentioning also that the size of her tip would reflect her insensitivity. Then, halfway through the meal, we encountered a dilemma when Misti had to go to the rest room. Taking the wheelchair back the hall toward the ladies' room, we realized that a cigarette machine was blocking the hallway, cutting down on the room to maneuver the wheelchair. Once again, our friends came to the rescue, placing Misti across their clasped arms, a human swing carrying her into the rest room. Two women already in the room glared as our heroes entered the ladies' room, but by this time, I was brooking no interference from anyone who was insensitive, unimaginative, or just plain rude. Just let them complain, I steamed to myself, now on guard against any muttered remarks. After all, this was a public restaurant, and the managers had the nerve to put a handicapped parking place in front without offering decent access to a table or the rest rooms.

As we left the restaurant, the manager approached us and told us that, should we want to bring Misti back, we were welcome to use the restaurant's delivery door, which has no steps. I thanked him and explained about the cigarette machine in the hall and the inaccessibility to the rest room. The look on his face revealed that he had no idea that the vending machine could have caused such an inconvenience. Apologizing profusely, he begged us to come back and give them another chance.

◎

Tuesday brought an unexpected surprise as Heather and Rani, having skipped school for the day, appeared in the hall. Misti was terribly excited to let them in on the details of her recent outing, communicating in a combination of sign and sound. Listening and watching, I came to the startling realization that graduation was only forty-six days ahead. Though Misti had certainly made great strides, the time did not seem long enough to allow her to accomplish the dream of leaving the Rehab and attending graduation services at Mercersburg Academy. But as I listened to the encouragement these two loyal friends gave her, I realized that even this might be a possibility.

Discussion with the team dampened our hopes—six weeks was not much time—but then, I realized, the team had never promised anything specific. Even the doctors, who seemed generally pleased with Misti's progress, had never held out the kind of hope necessary to allow us all to dream of a truly good future for Misti. Perhaps they were afraid of disappointing their patients and their patients' families; perhaps they could not stand to disappoint themselves if greater rehabilitation proved impossible. Or perhaps the answer was simpler: In these litigious days, perhaps most medical professionals are afraid of being sued by people if they give hope that never comes to fruition. Still, the fact remained that without being offered any specific medical hope, Misti had come this far.

One thing was becoming clear: whether or not she made it to the Mercersburg graduation, the time was approaching when Misti would no longer need the in-patient care of the Rehab, even though she would continue to need therapy. Despite Misti's undeniable progress, however, the Bryn Mawr team was fearful of the future if Misti were to return to Waynesboro. There, she had an awful lot of friends who would stop in for a visit, then buzz off with a cheery, "Good-bye, Misti. Gotta go, there's a party," and Misti, unable to accompany them, would realize her deficits too soon and become depressed enough to give up. According to the experts, this could even cause her to regress. In any case, they said, she could not continue to improve without all the therapies she was undertaking at Bryn Mawr. Going home to Waynesboro would mean that she would discontinue the horseback riding, warm-water therapy, and other therapies that were technical and difficult to duplicate off-site.

The team suggested that I keep the townhouse in Chesterbrook, or even better, look for a one-story house with wheelchair access and continue living in Paoli, bringing Misti back to Bryn Mawr each day for continued therapy until she had reached her full potential. But when I questioned what her full potential was, they would not offer me any concrete hope that the situation would someday be better than it was at present. And there were further questions. Staying at or near Bryn Mawr would mean further separation from the family—and at great personal and financial cost. How much longer could we go on the way we had been, with Misti and me hours from Harry and the rest of the family, trying to keep going in unfamiliar surroundings? And how could we continue to afford a separate house with monthly rental while continuing to pay for the necessary therapies?

I went back to Chesterbrook that night with my head spinning. What would happen if Misti left Bryn Mawr? What if she were to stay? What if I simply didn't listen to the experts? I believed she could make a fuller recovery. But where was my expertise in this area? Who was I to hold such hopes? After all, these good-hearted professionals who had worked with Misti for months now were experts, had seen brain trauma day after day, patient after patient, while I had had only this one experience. Perhaps my maternal instincts and hopes were clouding my better judgment, keeping me from facing reality. But how could I abandon my dreams for Misti now, when she herself so clearly shared them, too?

I drifted off to sleep that night with conflicting thoughts chasing themselves around in my tired head. Should we stay in the area? Could I take the chance and defy the experts, trusting that Misti could continue to recover even if we did not stay near Bryn Mawr? One of my questions was answered when I picked up the mail the next morning. In it was a notice that the town house had been sold and I would have to leave by May 2.

Sitting in the Rehab's cafeteria later that day, I was joined by one of the Bryn Mawr social workers. She had always been helpful with decisions in the past, and my hope was that she would have something to offer this time. After I explained the situation to her, she reminded me of the condo we owned in Ocean City, Maryland. If it was unwise for Misti to go back to regular life in Waynesboro so quickly, perhaps we could use the condo as an interim site for her continued recovery. This solution would not be without its problems, but I felt sure it had real possibilities.

Once again energized and hopeful, I went back to Misti's room. There, at the large black board, I drew two palm trees and in the same script that appears on the front of the condo complex wrote "Palm Bay." Misti was clearly puzzled. As she tried to figure out what I had written and why, I asked her to try to remember. But from the blank look in her eyes, it was clear that she had no idea what "Palm Bay" might be.

But there was no more time for depression and worry that day. Therapies went on as usual, and when Harry arrived in the afternoon, we took Misti out to a local restaurant for dinner, then out to a nearby shopping center to buy her new bibs and jeans, three sizes smaller than those she had worn before the accident. Her body was so frail and small that it was hard to believe her thin legs had once danced ballet.

Harry had to leave at 9:00 P.M., but he returned the following morning at 10:00 A.M.—six hours of driving in under twenty-four hours. A few days later, he had to return home. Long before, he had made arrangements to take a fishing trip to Canada with an old buddy from Waynesboro. He could not really help here, and I feared that we were hitting a wall, that rather than buoying each other with optimism, we were starting to sink each other with worry. He really needed some time away to clear his mind.

In the gym for Misti's physical therapy a few days later, I sat down beside a sweet-looking woman in a wheelchair who I had seen often in the Rehab's various therapy rooms. She asked how Misti was doing, and, when she heard about our dilemma, she reached into a pocket and pulled out the keys to her home, located only about ten minutes from Bryn Mawr Rehab. She told me that she wanted me to use her home when I had to move from Chesterbrook, since she would be at the Rehab for another month yet and the house was standing empty. She told me that she had watched me with Misti each day, and that she wanted to help in any way she could. To think that a stranger would give me the keys to her house and trust me to live there! I accepted with gratitude, knowing that not only were my worries about finding a new place much eased but also that I would be living even closer to the Rehab. I looked at the keys and thought that although the woman's name might be Barbara Lewis, she was really an angel in a wheelchair.

Over the weekend, a friend from Waynesboro arrived with her husband's pickup truck to help me move the clothes, books, plants, and other personal items I had accumulated in the past months to Barbara Lewis's home. After completing this errand, I went to get Misti and take her out to dinner. She had come to enjoy eating out; she always did her very best not to make a mess at the table and put a great deal of effort into speaking clearly so that the waitresses could understand her. At the same time, I always made a point of repeating her order casually, as if in passing—"Oh, Misti, a hamburger sounds great, but I'm going to have a chef salad myself. Do you think I should order fries, too, or can we share an order?" In this way, I tried to make sure that we didn't have a repeat of that first unfortunate incident. Misti was working so hard: She did not need to be embarrassed for her efforts.

We celebrated Harry's birthday without him while he was off on his well-earned fishing trip in Canada. Misti had made him a card on the computer and mailed it to him. Tonight's outing would be the first time it would be just the two of us, and I was a little nervous, but it was time I got comfortable at taking Misti out alone. If we moved to Ocean City for the summer, I would need to do many things for her alone.

Not remembering the problems with the vending machine in the hall outside the bathroom, Misti decided we should go to the Crab Shanty once again. But by the time we were ready to go, a spring downpour was underway, and getting to the car while pushing a wheelchair and holding an umbrella over the two of us proved to be quite a task. At the restaurant, I was relieved to see that the handicapped parking place was available, even though it was located nowhere near the delivery entrance without steps that the manager had suggested we use. Once I got us inside, we laughed at our drenched hair and clothes and prepared to enjoy ourselves. Misti had made great progress with eating and swallowing and was excited about ordering real food. I cut it up as small as possible and she concentrated on chewing it very well.

It was still pouring as we got ready to leave. I hurried to get Misti into the car and the wheelchair into the trunk. Then, as I approached the driver's side of the car, I heard her laughter—the same eerie, animal-like laugh she had produced before when overexcited or overtired. It was impossible to calm her down; she just laughed and laughed, hysterically, seemingly at nothing. Finally, pointing to the windshield, she said, "Arrested." Stepping out into the rain to remove the paper from the windshield, I realized that Misti was right. We had been given a citation for parking in the handicapped space without a permit. I told her that I would go to the police station tomorrow and explain to them that we had had a wheelchair and everything would be okay, and her laughter finally subsided.

In the morning, I went to the police station and tried to explain what had happened, but they were adamant that I pay the seventy-five-dollar fine. There would be no exceptions; without a handicapped license or a handicapped card on my dash in the car, they said, I had parked illegally. They said they had to be stern because many people who are not handicapped use such parking spots for their convenient location, especially when the weather is bad. In vain I explained that I would never do such a thing, that I did not realize that people would use a space reserved for handicapped people if they didn't need it, but I was told that ignorance of the law was no excuse and that I must pay the fine.

When I recounted the story back at Bryn Mawr, I learned that the staff were well aware of the regulations regarding handicapped license and parking permits. Why couldn't they have mentioned this when I signed the permission slip to take Misti out? More importantly, what kind of a mixed-up world fines a careless driver only forty dollars for causing an accident that leaves my daughter handicapped and yet charges me nearly twice that amount for using the handicapped space to take care of her? In physical therapy, Misti had just been fitted for new shoes with special lifts to allow for better balance control. The seventy-five dollars I'd just paid would have made a nice dent in that bill, I reflected sourly.

Nine

As May wore on, Misti continued to make progress, but because she lacked insight into her condition and the deficits the accident had left her with, there wasn't much agreement about where she would go once she was released in June. The atmosphere at the next team meeting grew heated as we talked about whether Misti would be able to attend the Mercersburg graduation, then rose to fever pitch when the discussion moved on to the subject of my taking her to Ocean City for the summer. Everyone in the room, except for the Aetna nurse, Ann Diller, and myself, thought this would be a bad idea.

We were warned that away from the Rehab, it would be difficult to find proper therapists, that there would be difficulties in finding space for the therapies to take place, that we'd have to locate a lab to have the necessary blood tests done each week to check Misti's Tegretol level. How would we find a doctor who knew enough about brain trauma to be able to understand Misti's situation and advise us? Could I coordinate all of this? I had no answer to these questions and at that point did not know even where to start looking. Most of all, a deep, hidden fear ate at me: Maybe they were right. Maybe I would not be up to the challenge. Maybe Misti would not recover further no matter what we did or where we went. Confused and tired, I went back to Misti's room.

The phone was ringing when I arrived, and I answered it to hear my sister-in-law Beck's excited voice, telling me that she had just read an ad in the Hagerstown, Maryland, newspaper for something called Alternatives in Community Treatments (ACT), a private community group that helped families who had been hit by injury or ill health coordinate treatments and find programs that could keep family members out of institutions. She was not sure the organization could help me, but it might at least provide a lead. When I dialed the number Beck gave me, a man answered and introduced himself as Bill Burlin. We discussed Misti's situation for a few minutes, and then he suggested that I "stop in to see them for further discussion." As it turned out, he was only a short distance from the Rehab, and we arranged that he would come to Bryn Mawr to meet me the following day. Shaking a little in nervous anticipation, I told Misti that we might be on to something.

After the phone call, Misti told me that she knew what the "Palm Bay" on the chalkboard meant: "It is the name of the street we live on in

Ocean City." I told her that the name of our street in Ocean City was Bayshore Drive and that she would have to think some more. She stared intently at the board, obviously thinking hard. She no longer looked blank, as she had when I first put the words on the board; she seemed to recognize them now, but was clearly having trouble fitting these pieces of the puzzle into their proper places. In all the talking I had done when she was in the coma, I had certainly told her about the condo, including the name on the building and the colors it was painted. It was as though she had retained a lot of what I had told her—or she had the information stored somewhere in deep, long-term memory—but was having difficulty sorting the information in her brain. I had a mental image of a file cabinet that had been overturned. All the files were still there, but not yet in any order that could be used. Some of them may even have fallen to the bottom of the cabinet where they were inaccessible. When I discussed this image with Dr. Audieh, she agreed that this was a rather elegant analogy of what had happened to Misti's brain and memory—and a much clearer explanation than any offered by the medical professionals or researchers who worked with brain trauma all the time.

The next item on the agenda was getting an authorized handicapped parking card to prevent further parking fines or confrontations with the police. This proved to be a greater feat than I ever imagined. The police department—which was, after all, located near a major rehabilitation facility and must have been used to such requests—insisted that I bring Misti into the local station to prove that she was in fact handicapped. Worse, they insisted that I get her to the station—and up the five steep steps in front—between the hours of 9:00 A.M. and 4:00 P.M., thereby sacrificing precious therapy hours, which the Rehab was loathe to allow. This was really an impossible request, as I tried to explain, but once again I was told that "rules are rules." When I asked the policeman why he could not come out to Bryn Mawr and see Misti for himself, he insisted that this was not the way things were done. For a while, we were at a most frustrating impasse. Eventually, I persuaded the authorities to watch one of the videos I'd made of Misti at the Rehab, and they finally issued the handicapped card.

When I arrived back at Bryn Mawr, it was time to meet Bill Burlin, who had brought a young woman he introduced as Cathy Cosgrove, one of the case coordinators for ACT. The meeting was a real success. They were eager to help and, though not sure how easy it would be to find places to conduct the therapies in Ocean City, they were positive that we could find good therapists from among the many young people who spend the summers in the resort town. They promised to start the search and get back to me in a few days. In the meantime, Misti had continued to make progress, saying excitedly, "Palm Bay, I know what it is, it is the name of our condo." She then spelled out some numbers. I did not recognize them immediately, but soon recalled they were the numbers keyed to the security system at our home in Waynesboro. Clearly the information had been somewhat misfiled, but we were all thrilled to know she was still a whiz with numbers.

Sunday was Mothers' Day and Misti had planned to show me a great day. Harry helped her make reservations at a nice local restaurant, and accompanied by Max, we all went out to dinner. Though both Max and Harry were happy at Misti's continued progress, I suspected that their feelings were coming from two very different perspectives: With the innocence and air of invulnerability of youth, Max was sure that it was only a matter of time before Misti was back to being the girl he'd fallen in love with, while Harry, having taken in and finally accepted how much brain damage she'd sustained, was both astonished and grateful at just how far she had come. In the back of my mind was what Max's mother had told me about how frustrated Max was, how he used a punching bag continuously when he was home; I wondered how long even the most loyal of young men could take the pressure the accident had placed on their relationship.

As the month went on and Misti was doing more work in crafts therapy and on the computer in cognitive retraining, it was clear that her new glasses were not doing the trick and that we would have to consult another eye doctor. The new ophthalmologist thought that there was quite a bit of damage to muscles and nerves in the back of the eyes; however, he did not think that there was anything major that could be done to correct that damage. Since that was the case, he felt the glasses she already had worked about as well as any would. This was most frustrating. It was clear that Misti's progress in a number of areas was being stymied by the fact that she could not see as well as she might have.

Though Misti had by this time accepted that she had more rehab to do physically—that her ability to move her arms and legs had been affected by the accident—she did not recognize that she had any mental deficits stemming from the accident. She never really seemed to connect the brain and nerve injuries she'd sustained to her mental abilities, and she insisted that she could still do everything mentally that she could have before—set her own daily schedule, graduate from Mercersburg, go on to college, etc. Of course, we didn't want to discourage her hopes and dreams for fear that she would just give up, but we all knew that she had in fact sustained mental damage. For example, she could not remember anything about wanting to be a doctor or even the Mercersburg Academy subjects in which she had once made honors grades. Sadly, I recalled the afternoon I'd spent composing letters to the colleges—Georgetown, Loyola, Gettysburg, and Washington and Lee— that had eagerly accepted Misti and even offered her scholarship aid. I'd had to tell them about the accident and let them know that Misti wouldn't be coming after all.

The psychological and psychiatric evaluations done at Bryn Mawr in May put Misti's intelligence at a fourth-grade level and her emotional maturity at about that of a three-year-old. And because brain trauma is such an unpredictable phenomenon, there was no way anyone could offer realistic hope that the situation would improve. Even though Misti was making progress, there was no long-term treatment plan or scheme: Each week we all would see what Misti could do and let that guide us toward what she might try to do next.

Whatever Misti's current emotional age and our hopes of further progress, it became obvious that her emotional makeup had been damaged. When Harry was taking his leave of her one night, an emotionally exhausted Misti started in with that eerie laughter once again. Doctor Audieh was now sure that Misti had lost the ability to cry when she was sad, and that for the present, at least, she could only express that feeling with the strange, inappropriate laughter. And since Misti had no idea that her reactions were inappropriate and was having difficulties with short-term memory to boot, it really wasn't possible at this point for any kind of insight-oriented emotional therapy to take place. That would have to wait until further recovery had taken place. All we could do was watch, wait, and hope that this would prove to be a phase we'd all get through quickly.

Meanwhile, since Misti seemed to be making progress on all other fronts, we decided to move forward in the areas of personal grooming, such as hair-combing and toothbrushing, that I'd been helping her with. The idea was that Misti would learn to do more for herself, such as bathing herself with the aid of a new shower chair. As I watched her propel her wheelchair down the hall toward the shower room, I realized that she had fulfilled my early prayers for recovering some mobility. But as a human being and as her mother, I now wanted so much more for her: I wanted her to be able to care for herself, to get back to school, to have a home of her own, a family, an education.

With every step forward, every bit of progress, we learned there were new and unexpected phases of recovery. After an excursion to a nearby mall with Harry and Max, for instance, Misti was very irritable for the next several days. She explained that all the girls at the mall had been staring at Max and obviously wondering why such a good-looking young man was with someone who looked like her—thin, pale, in a wheelchair, with her head falling to one side as she tired. When we tried to comfort her and dispute her reasoning—after all, we pointed out, Max had chosen to be with her—she started to kick and hit us, then laughed her eerie laugh. It was small comfort indeed to know that Misti's fears, dawning self-consciousness at her physical state, and faulty reasoning were part of brain trauma and the recovery process.

A day later, Misti seemed to have calmed down substantially, and we started to talk seriously about the possibility of her attending Mercersburg's graduation. There seemed to be at least a chance that she would be able to go, though the situation was touch and go until the very end. The Rehab staff was afraid that she would not be able to handle seeing other, "normal" kids without suffering a major setback. I worried that the students who hadn't seen Misti since the accident would be shocked at her appearance and make her uncomfortable and self-conscious. But those concerns would have to wait. In the meantime, we went shopping for the customary white graduation dress. Max had reminded Misti of the white dress she had purchased back in January for the prom sponsored by his school, but that was far too formal for the graduation ceremony. Now, however, the thought of the prom gown hanging at home in the closet agitated Misti. In fact, she was so upset—the weird canned laughter was back, accompanied by hitting and kicking—at the idea of missing the prom that we came up with an alternative plan: a formal night out for Misti and Max. Max and his parents made plans to come up dressed in evening clothes; Harry and I decided we would do the same, and the six of us would all go out to dinner.

The latest stage of recovery was proving difficult. It wasn't just that Misti wasn't reasoning well or having odd emotional reactions to daily events. In addition, she was actively confabulating, borrowing from movies, TV shows, and other people's experiences to tell stories or make accusations that couldn't possibly be true. For instance, after she began attending group meetings with other patients, all of them brain injured, Misti began to confuse the stories that other group members had told and became convinced that they had happened to her. The staff was well aware of the possibility of brain trauma patients confusing their own situations with those from stories or movies; this was why they allowed only certain television shows and movies to be shown at the Rehab and why the viewing of soap operas were strictly forbidden, even for long-time fans like Misti. From my vantage point—behind a one-way window through which I could observe the meetings—it seemed that some of the same problems arose from the patient group social meetings. The patients, many of whom were without emotional or behavioral inhibitions as a result of their disabilities, discussed sex freely, often it seemed, trying to outdo one another in the wildness of their tales. When patients dwelled on the subject of sex for too long, the staff members running the meeting would try to change the topic and call on patients who hadn't been heard from in a while. Interestingly, though there were more men than women in the groups, the women were not at all reticent about talking about sexual fantasies or imaginings; one woman in particular was convinced she was irresistible to men and talked on and on of seductions that couldn't have taken place—they weren't physically possible. The staff accepted that the talk of seduction and sexual acting out were stages of recovery and were both nonjudgmental and vigilant so that no one could be hurt.

However, everything Misti observed, deduced, and imagined *seemed* very real to her and could upset her greatly. For instance, she put together the fact that Max was not staying with her at the Rehab at night with the fact that he was staying with me at Chesterbrook, often without Harry or his parents being present, and then came to the "logical" conclusion that we were sleeping together. When I asked about Misti's confabulations, the staff said once again that this was a phase of coming out, but had no new answers or advice for me. The whole situation—Misti's wild imaginings, her obvious increased interest in sex with decreased inhibitions, and her close proximity to other patients with the same problems—scared me to death. I was very concerned about her continued attendance at the overstimulating group meetings and later wondered whether many of the problems we later had could have been avoided had Misti not been exposed to the problems of others at that point. In fact, I tried as often as I could to keep Misti from going to the meetings, but the Bryn Mawr staff felt that they were essential for greater patient socialization, since all of the patients needed to relearn how to get along with people in the real world. I went along with this Bryn Mawr strategy somewhat reluctantly because I was scared for Misti. Yes, she needed to get used to being with other people again, but why not try for a wider group than the patients at the Rehab? While I'm not sure I actually prayed more at this stage, I sure kept the line to God open and talked with him just about every waking hour.

Accompanying the beginning of this trying phase was the news that Misti might now be entering into a state of depression, common in patients with brain or spinal cord injuries who have started to realize the extent of their disabilities. No one suggested Misti take antidepressants, probably because of the difficulties and dangers of mixing Tegretol with other drugs. Again, there were no real answers, just suggestions of waiting and promises of vigilance.

At the next team meeting, one of the psychiatrists, Dr. Armstrong, suggested that since she was making so much physical progress, we should focus on the possibility of Misti's moving to the Laurels, the independent living section of the Rehab, before she left Bryn Mawr in mid-June. The purpose of the independent living unit, which was separate from the main Rehab building, was to prepare patients for life outside the Rehab. In the Laurels, Dr. Armstrong explained to Misti, she would have her own room and the responsibility for keeping it neat; she would also have to help prepare food, clean up after meals, and do her own laundry; and she had to get herself up to the main building for therapy. From the therapies she had undergone within the Rehab proper, it was clear that Misti could manage these tasks, but her preoccupation with sexual matters was still a source of great worry.

In fact, as the time for the planned move to the Laurels neared, Misti began to talk of sex almost all the time. If Max loved her, she said, he would show it by making love to her. Dr. Armstrong became alarmed at continuing reports from other doctors, assistants, therapists, as well as male patients, about being propositioned by Misti. Though not unexpected, the intensity of Misti's conversation and behavior concerned all of us; there would be much less security at the Laurels than in the rest of the Rehab, and since it would be their responsibility to keep Misti safe, the Bryn Mawr staff were at least as concerned as I was. They knew quite well the difficulties involved: Many of the other patients would have no better judgment than Misti and putting them together would have been adding gasoline to an already smoldering fire.

In short order, it became obvious to all of us that the move to the Laurels would have to be postponed. Dr. Armstrong explained to Misti that she just wasn't yet ready for the Laurels, and though Misti was eager to get out of the protected unit and out to the wider world, she seemed to accept this. Curiously, though she could be strong-minded on occasion, Misti did not focus on the problems of being restrained or on the practical matters of day-to-day living. She liked to get away from the Rehab buildings, out into the air, out in the car, but she had no real concept of how impaired she still was physically or how difficult it would be for her to function in the world. Watching Misti to see that no one took advantage of her vulnerability had become a full-time job—and one that was interrupted for me only by very strange circumstances.

As I was walking to the car one morning with some of Misti's clothes over my arm, balancing an umbrella, I started to feel odd, almost as though I was looking through the water of a fish bowl. As I got nearer to the car, the feeling got worse and I realized I was going to pass out. My lungs could not take in enough air and I watched my hand in slow motion trying to grab the fender of the car. When I opened my eyes somewhat later, all the clothes I'd been carrying or wearing were wet and cars were whizzing by on the highway. I am not a small person, yet no one seemed to see me. I knew I had to get up off the wet ground, but my head hurt, and everything was spinning. When I touched my forehead, I realized that rain was mixing with blood and running down my face. Returning to the house for dry clothes, I looked into the mirror and saw that my forehead had a small cut and brush burn.

Since I was now late in getting to the Rehab, I hurried back to the car and drove the wet roads to Bryn Mawr. Once there, I realized I was an hour and a half behind schedule, so I ran ahead to physical therapy and picked up Misti to go on to cognitive retraining therapy. In the hall, I met Aunt Goldie and Uncle Ora, who had with them Meme Semler and Dave and Beck's youngest daughter, Jenny. Aunt Goldie greeted me with, "God, you look bad." Though I felt lousy and was annoyed at Goldie's bluntness, I didn't argue or explain what had just happened. I was sure the episode was not a big deal and that I'd be fine. They inquired about Harry's whereabouts, and I explained that he would arrive on Saturday, which was planned as Misti's and Max's formal night.

Thankful that it had stopped raining, at noon we all took Misti out for equestrian therapy. The family enjoyed watching her on the horse, and, after a very enjoyable afternoon, we stopped for pizza on the way back to Bryn Mawr. On arriving back at the Rehab, however, Misti was obviously overtired or overexcited or both and had one of her laughing spells. This left a number of the family in tears, unable to understand how we could possibly say that Misti was recovering under the circumstances.

After getting Misti to bed, I returned home, strangely exhausted. But sleep did not come easy, and I dialed our number in Waynesboro to leave Harry a reminder about bringing his tux when he came up for the weekend. When Harry arrived at the Rehab, I told him about my fainting experience in the parking lot, and he insisted that I see a doctor. Feeling sure that there was no real problem, I consented to go to Paoli Hospital and get checked out, but put it off until morning. To my surprise, when I went into the emergency room the next day, the doctor promptly admitted me to the cardiac unit, attached a Holter heart monitoring device, and ordered me not to get out of bed. I was very upset because the next evening was Misti's formal night out, which she had been looking forward to for weeks; this could not happen now. But no amount of begging would make them let me out. If I had known this would happen, I would not have come, but I'd come to the hospital to get checked out, and there I stayed. Harry assured me that he would represent the family for both of us, that the important thing was for us to find out what had made me faint.

The next day, Max and his family arrived for the formal night, Max with flowers for Misti. I was thankful I had already ordered a boutonniere for her to give him. Before they went out to dinner, Harry, Misti, Max, and his parents came to the hospital to see me. I was sorry to miss the occasion, but I felt wonderful seeing Misti looking so beautiful in her white prom gown. The next day, Harry reported that the evening had been a great success and that he would be responsible for helping Misti move to the Laurels the next day. Meanwhile, Chuck and Teresa made the trip up from Waynesboro to visit me, bringing Victor and Valera along.

After a week in the hospital, with lots of bed rest and many tests, the doctors decided that I had been suffering from arrhythmia of the heart brought on by stress. With promises of behavior modification on my part, they finally released me. Fortunately, the next two weeks were much easier than the previous weeks had been. Misti's transfer to the Laurels proved good for both of us. She heeded what her counselors said about the tasks she had to undertake there, and they helped her adjust to her new, more responsibility-oriented lifestyle. At the beginning, the transition went more easily than I had anticipated, which left time for me to follow doctors' orders.

A few days later, I watched proudly as Misti was loaded into a van equipped to take patients for outings and drove off with some of them to the local pizza parlor. I knew that the Rehab staff were concerned that I would find it hard to disengage from Misti when the time came because of our closeness and her recent dependence on me, but in my heart, I knew they were wrong. When she could walk away from me and go off to college, I told myself, I would cry, but they would be tears of joy, not sadness. If she could not walk but left with the aid of appliances or in a chair, I told myself, I would still be ecstatic to see her go. In the back of my mind, I knew that it would be hard, but everything I was doing was for her, and my real reward would be getting Misti back and seeing her launched into the world.

When she returned from the outing, Misti was tired and began laughing that terrible laughter I had heard so many times before. I offered another prayer that this phase would soon pass also. After listening to her describe the trip with the group to get pizza, I realized she was scared and could not fully understand why she was out with all these handicapped people. It was evident that until she was loaded into the van with the group, she had never seen herself as truly handicapped. Maybe her refusal to accept her handicaps would ultimately prove to be for the good, making her work harder to recover, but for the present, it was a burden.

After getting Misti to bed, I had to head out to find my new home. While I had been in the hospital, Harry had moved my belongings to a hotel; Barbara Lewis had recovered enough to come home, and I was once again nomadic. Since the idea of going to the Laurels was for Misti to learn to do more on her own, I had to stay out of her way, and I found myself with an unaccustomed amount of time on my hands. I quickly decided to spend some of my time back in the main Rehab building with the other patients. Maybe, I thought, I could learn something from them that would help me later with Misti; if nothing else, I could provide some companionship to some very lonely people whose families were unable to visit often.

In the two weeks that Misti was in the Laurels, I learned to talk with patients who could only communicate with the use of computer devices on the tray attached to their chairs. I spent one day with a young man who slowly, but accurately, hit one key, then another, and another on the keyboard. He spelled out each word he wanted to share with me at the rate of perhaps three letters per minute. One of the nurses explained to me that the device he used was called a facilitated communicator. He was obviously terribly proud to be able to talk to anyone who could take the time to "listen," to sit endlessly with him while he painstakingly got out just one short sentence. I knew that although the staff spent as much time with him as possible, he was very lonely. My heart went out to this intelligent fellow who had had the misfortune to fall asleep at the wheel one night and run off the road, lying unconscious for hours until someone discovered the accident and called for help. Looking into his clear blue eyes, I had the feeling he understood more than he could express, but I would never know how much.

Toward the end of the next week, Max called to say that he wanted to come up to Paoli for the Memorial Day weekend, but that no hotel would rent to a young person who wanted to stay without his parents. I coaxed the manager of my hotel into renting me a second room across the hall from mine and then phoned Brenda to tell her that Max could come up and stay the weekend.

Memorial Day weekend would be a wonderful opportunity to take Misti out overnight—a necessary step to get her used to the world outside Bryn Mawr—but it was not going to be easy to get this accomplished because the outing would require the consent of the entire Bryn Mawr staff, including doctors, nurses, and therapists, each of whom had a slightly different opinion about the possible effects on Misti's future rehabilitation. Finally, however, permission came through, and Max and I took an excited Misti to our hotel. Thus, Misti was able to celebrate the summer's first holiday the same way as many other people—lounging beside the pool. However, the overnight stay proved harder than I had anticipated. I had not realized all the difficulties of using a wheelchair in a hotel room, especially the bathroom; the tub and shower proved to be too much for either of us to handle, and Misti had to settle for a sponge bath. The next day, Bonnie and Rani Carniello came by the hotel to visit. The day was perfect, and, in the evening after our guests had gone, I returned Misti to the Laurels. Apparently neither overtired nor overexcited, she went to sleep calmly and happily, counting the days until she would be out for good.

As time sped toward mid-June and ACT made arrangements for the therapies and equipment necessary for our stay in Ocean City, Misti seemed more like herself—except for her sexual acting out. Jokingly, I told her one day that her morals were those of an alley cat. I was stunned at her vehemence and nearly violent response. Looking at me with true hatred, more than I had ever seen in her, she screamed haltingly, "I hate you, bitch, I hate you." The words tore through my heart sharply; I could not believe that my daughter had stammered out the words. Stunned, I next heard her spit out venomously, "I hope you die, you f—-ing bitch, I hope you die." It was impossible to talk to her, to tell her I'd been teasing, and I found myself heading back to the hotel, tears burning my eyes as I drove. What had I done to make her act like this?

In the flash of an eye, our short "honeymoon" period had ended and we were into an excruciatingly uncomfortable new stage. For the next week, I did not hear one decent word from Misti. Again and again, the staff reassured me that her hostile language and attitude were yet another stage recovering coma patients experience, but I flinched every time I heard the words that poured from her mouth. I had heard the expression, "cussing like a sailor," but I had certainly never imagined that it would apply to Misti. But suddenly, everything had become a struggle, every conversation provoked a verbal rebellion replete with words I had seldom heard before. One day she insisted that she needed six hundred dollars to buy Max a gift. No amount of talk could sway her. She wanted the money and I'd better get it or she would kill me, she said. She was small and physically almost powerless, but her words and the tone they were spoken in were absolutely chilling.

Her remarkable change in attitude had the Laurels' counselors and the Bryn Mawr doctors seriously considering changing their minds about authorizing Misti's discharge from the Rehab the next week. Given her sudden hostility to me and the strength she was likely to gain as she recovered, they were very concerned that I might not be able to handle her alone. They felt that the weekend's excursion away from the protection of the Rehab had caused this change in attitude, which scared me much more than I let on. The clawing doubt was back: Maybe they were right. Maybe the best thing to do would be for me to find a place to stay near Bryn Mawr and take Misti back for therapy each day. But then, of course, I'd still be alone with her at night.

Again, I called on God for guidance. Since he seemed to be the only one who listened to me with any consistency, I now complained to him about the unfairness of life. I told him that I was nearing the end of my tether, that I feared I would soon be out of resources; again I questioned why this had happened. But the answer, as before, remained clear: "Why not?" And I had to trust that God would once again get us through the next phase. Then I dropped face down into the bed and slept dreamlessly.

The next morning, I woke refreshed and strangely confident. Drawing on reserves I hadn't known I had, I assured the worried Rehab team that I could in fact handle the move to Ocean City without problem, that I understood that Misti's bad language was just another stage on the way to recovery, that I had watched other patients go through it, and that I would watch over Misti and not let her attitude, her language, or her antics get to me. As I packed the car for the long anticipated Mercersburg graduation weekend, which Misti had been given the green light to attend at last, I came to the conclusion that if the Bryn Mawr staff had enough faith in my ability to handle this, then I certainly should not doubt myself. Everything would be fine once I got her out of the Rehab. And once we were home or at Ocean City, I would have help from Harry, too.

As we drove toward Waynesboro the next day—we were going to stop overnight at home before the Mercersburg festivities—I talked to Misti about the upcoming baccalaureate service, observing that her teachers and friends, especially her beloved Mr. Jones, the school's chaplain, would be glad to see her and so proud of her if she did not use bad language. At Exit 3 in Greencastle, Misti suddenly asked me to stop. She looked hard in both directions and asked if this was the way home or to school. If we turned right, I told her, we would go straight to Mercersburg and be at the Academy in about fifteen minutes. But, if we turned left and went through the Square, we would be home in about fifteen minutes. She was deep in thought, and I wondered whether she was remembering life before the accident or whether she was trying to put together images pulled from my endless monologues when she was coming out of the coma. The fact that she recognized anything was a real victory.

Now very curious and hopeful, I made the rest of the drive into a quiz: Each time we approached a street that we should turn onto, I asked if she knew which way to go, but she could not figure anything out until we were in Waynesboro near Rani's house, when she asked me to stop. I came to a stop at the curb just in front of the Carniellos' house, at which Misti sat staring intently. She seemed to have some memories, but it still took several minutes before she reconnected with the fact that this was where Rani lived. As we drove away, she looked very serious as she said, "I think we have to turn left." We took the left and she repeated the same thing once again, and then, as we took the second left onto Ringgold Street, my heart leaped. The old oak tree in front of our house was covered in yellow ribbons, literally hundreds of yellow ribbons. Helium-filled balloons flew in front of the house and there was a banner welcoming Misti home—truly a sight to behold. Rani was there to welcome us as well as many other friends and neighbors. Inside the house were flowers from neighbors and relatives. That night, for the first time in months, we slept in our own beds.

The baccalaureate was the only activity scheduled for the following day. In the service for graduates, faculty, families, and friends, Mr. Jones told of the accident and how Misti had fought to cheat death and return to the school to be with everyone for this event. A collection was taken during the ceremony and the proceeds were given to Misti for anything she might need in her recovery. After the moving ceremony, we went to Misti's dorm room to collect as much of Misti's stuff as possible to take home. Odette came home with us to spend one last night with her roommate. Tomorrow their lives would part, perhaps forever. Odette's father would arrive from Africa to take her back home, and one could only wonder when they would ever see each other again.

On Saturday morning, Aunt Goldie, Uncle Ora, Meme Ray and Meme Semler, Chuck, Teresa, Cork, Jill, Emily and Brenda, Anthony, and Max accompanied us to the graduation at Mercersburg. We all knew that Misti would not receive a Mercersburg diploma at the ceremony; despite her high grades and many credits, the school would not bend its strict requirements for her. Instead she would receive a certificate stating that she was a member of the class of 1988. Perhaps next year, as her recovery continued, she would be able to fulfill the requirements for classroom time at Mercersburg and receive an Academy diploma. For today, Max and a young man who was a member of the class carried the wheelchair up the few steps to the terrace where the outdoor ceremony took place.

Except for the fact that Misti was in a wheelchair wearing thick, dark glasses to protect her eyes, the day was as I had dreamed of it for the past several years. As the awards were given to outstanding students, however, it was almost impossible to hold back the tears. Misti surely would have received many of these awards if only she had not been cheated by the accident.

As the ceremony came to an end, Mr. Burgin, the headmaster, turned his back to the audience and addressed the class privately. It seemed clear that he was talking to them about Misti; many of the students looked her way and then moved to dry their eyes. The good-byes that day were very emotional.

After a family party—and another night in our own beds—we started on the trip back to Bryn Mawr. Except for a few isolated outbursts of rage and bad language, it had been a wonderful weekend.

Each June day now brought the end of Misti's stay at Bryn Mawr nearer. Cathy Cosgrove came up to Bryn Mawr and met with Harry and me to make all final arrangements for ongoing therapies in Ocean City. In the next ten days, she told us, she would have everything set up and ready for our arrival. The final week was filled with fittings for walkers and other items necessary for taking care of a handicapped person. At the last team meeting, the doctors, therapists, Cathy Cosgrove, and Ann Diller from Aetna all formally endorsed the plan for Misti to recover in Ocean City. Everyone agreed that Misti had come further than anyone could have ever dreamed or hoped, but the rehab staff also emphasized that Misti was now at a stage where going directly home would definitely be detrimental. Realizing her deficits before she could deal with them effectively would likely cause depression, which could tear down what had been built so carefully and patiently.

As a team, we decided that it would be beneficial for Misti's friends to make short visits, but not to talk of their plans at the beach. At this point, she could accept the idea that they had come to visit her and that they would be going home when they left; she would not be able to accept the idea that they would visit her and then go on to party or vacation elsewhere in Ocean City. But as long as her friends did not return to Bayshore Drive, she would have no way of knowing they were still in town and enjoying things that were not available to her.

On our last Saturday night in Paoli, Brenda, Anthony, Max, and his brother Stanley took Misti and me out to dinner to celebrate. We tried a new restaurant, which had steps in the front that led up to a porch. Rather than carry Misti in the wheelchair, Max picked her up, with Anthony and Stanley following with the chair. I watched in sheer horror as Max slipped and fell with Misti in his arms. Although she landed on top of him, her elbow hit the concrete with a sharp thud. Misti tried to assure us that she was all right, but as the evening went on, the joint started swelling noticeably.

Over dinner, we discussed the plans the Greys had made for Max to spend the summer in Ocean City to be near Misti. They had rented Max a condo about two blocks from ours. He would be required to get a job, but he would also be able to see Misti when he was not working. As they spoke, I had real doubts about the wisdom of these plans, and I ardently wished that Harry were here to talk this out with me. With all of Misti's anger toward me, her fears and jealousies about Max, her lack of sexual inhibition, and her continued need for intensive therapy, having Max around would probably be more difficult for everyone. Perhaps, I thought in great weariness, I should put my foot down and object, but I couldn't summon the energy. Maybe there would be a silver lining: Misti would have companionship from someone who understood the situation, and, since Max would be around, he might even be able to help with therapies and other practical matters. But that was my exhaustion speaking, not my heart and mind. When Harry arrived from Waynesboro about 11:00 P.M. that night, we discussed the situation. He, too, was apprehensive but felt there was little we could do since the Greys had already made the plans and had even rented the condo for Max. Further, Misti was sure to suffer a setback if her plans to see Max for the summer were upset now.

On Monday morning, the rehab staff told us that Misti had to go to Paoli Hospital for X-rays of her elbow, and we went along in the ambulance for the necessary tests. Unfortunately, the X-rays taken were not clear, and another set had to be taken the next day, delaying our departure for Ocean City. Misti did not take the news well, fearing that any delay would give Max an opportunity to go to Ocean City early, find another girlfriend, and forget her. Her reaction to the idea of more tests and possible treatment was extreme: She screamed and fought so strongly that she had to be restrained. Her cussing was back in full force, and she insisted that we should put her up for adoption since she did not want to be our daughter anymore. After the happiness of the baccalaureate and our relief at Misti's progress, this backsliding seemed very cruel. Tears fell from our eyes as she told us over and over how much she hated us and wished us both dead.

Cathy Cosgrove and Bill Burlin arrived the following morning to review with Misti the rules for living at the beach. Cathy would now be our contact with ACT, and she moved quickly to establish her authority, acutely aware that Misti must trust and respect it if this venture were to succeed. Cathy made it very clear that there would be definite limits on the time and duration of Max's visits. Though Misti agreed quite readily to abide by the rules, I was not at all sure that she would continue to follow the rules once we were in Maryland.

However, Cathy assured me that she and Bill had anticipated this very situation and decided on a strategy together. Though they were sure Misti would rebel later, the rules had to be set now; we would deal with Misti's rebellion and disobedience when it happened. Cathy added that she had spoken with Max on the subject and made it clear that if he did not help keep the rules, he would be forbidden to see Misti at all. From her past experience with other patients, Cathy now explained, she knew that we had a hard road ahead. She added that I must be used to this by now.

Even though I recognized that Cathy was probably right in her predictions, I didn't want to believe that the situation would be as difficult as she seemed to be anticipating. Instead, I told myself that things could only get better, that Ocean City would be wonderful, that the condo was the perfect place for Misti to complete her recovery, that everything would turn out well. After all, Misti had defied so many other predictions of disaster; other people were always anticipating the worst. Well, I knew my daughter, and I was certain that once again she would prove the experts wrong. Summer in Ocean City would work out just fine. As we were leaving the meeting room, I overheard one nurse tell another, "I do not know where that woman gets her guts, but if I ever get hurt, I want her on my side."

On Wednesday, just one day before Misti's scheduled discharge from Bryn Mawr, a brand-new wheelchair, which would leave Bryn Mawr with us, arrived. Misti was like a child with a new toy. Karen showed it to Misti in their final physical therapy session, before the last good-byes were said.

It was wonderful to be leaving Bryn Mawr for a new life, but also oddly sad. As Misti had emerged from the coma, she had bonded with the people at the Rehab and built a new life around the therapists and patients. The Laurels held a farewell party for Misti and another patient, Todd, who was very upset—not because he was leaving Bryn Mawr, but because his girlfriend had just broken up with him. This scenario was all too common for the Rehab's patients. Too often, once it was clear that a patient was no longer perfect, or would not completely heal, the love between the couple became one-sided. Sooner or later the one on the outside broke off the relationship. It was a sad fact of life.

One patient at the party was an exception to this rule. When Gregg came over to say good-bye to Misti and Todd, his wheelchair was being pushed by his mother, father, wife, and one-year-old son. His son had been an infant when Gregg was involved in an automobile accident that left him completely paralyzed and capable of making very little cognitive response to anyone. But throughout the year, his loving and loyal family had continued to make the daily trips to be with him. It was heartbreaking to watch the little boy sit on his unresponsive father's lap. My thoughts lingered: Maybe when people complain about how bad their everyday lives are, they should be forced to spend a week in a brain-trauma rehab.

On Thursday, June 16—131 days after the accident—we faced another stage in our new life. The discharge papers signed, each of the nurses hugged Misti and said good-bye. Every rehab has strict rules about nurses not becoming attached to their patients, but as Misti and Peggy embraced, it was clear that an exception had been made. Through teary eyes, I watched Misti say her farewells, thinking that she might cry at such an emotional moment. It was not to be, however. Her eyes stayed dry. She was still not able to cry. Perhaps Dr. Audieh was right; perhaps that emotion had been lost for Misti forever and she would never be able to feel that way again.

Though Misti was excited about going to Ocean City, a trip that would take us through Waynesboro, she seemed to have no memory of the drive we made only twelve days before. Her short- and perhaps medium-term memory continued to be impaired. At each turn I asked her if she knew where we should go next, but she had forgotten all the landmarks from the other trip. This time Misti did not seem to notice as we passed Rani's house and turned the familiar corner onto Ringgold Street. It was as though the entire expereince was new to her. Her eyes lit up only as we turned into the driveway to our home and she saw the forty-eight helium balloons flying over the house and the one hundred yellow ribbons on the old oak tree. Harry and Chuck and Cork and their families had made a large sign that covered the front of the house saying, "Good-bye, Bryn Mawr—Hello, Ocean City." After a festive barbecue dinner, we put a very tired Misti to bed in her own room.

The next day, we unpacked the tightly loaded car and put the winter clothes we had been wearing into the laundry room. Then we repacked summer clothes along with the necessary appliances—wheelchair, walker, commode rails—and started the next leg of our journey. Though we had discussed this trip for the last several weeks, Misti seemed very confused at all the changes, and I worried that we were making the move too fast. The problem was that we had no time to spare; we had to get ready to start therapies on Monday morning.

As we drove down Route 495 toward the beach, I continued to talk to Misti about all the changes she'd been through since February, and we decided to stop in Bethesda and let the nurses in the STU at Suburban Hospital see how well her recovery was coming along. As we entered the hospital, this time with me pushing Misti in a wheelchair, I felt the familiar dread of death, that feeling of sadness and despair. Even the smells were familiar. As we walked by the waiting room, the murmurs of a family waiting that eternal wait for news of their loved one brought back the memories of our being told, "If she lives another hour, there is a better chance." Sympathy flooded my soul as I passed the doorway, knowing that only God could do something for them at this terrible time.

We headed toward the large double swinging doors that separate the waiting families from the patients being cared for in the STU. I reached for the phone on the wall on the left side of the hall, saying that there was someone waiting to see the nurses. When they heard that it was Misti Morningstar, the doors swung open at once. Nurse Carolyn, still wearing the familiar ring of keys dangling from her shirt on the left shoulder, smiled and hugged Misti, and the other nurses followed suit. Each appreciatively noted how wonderful Misti looked and how far she had come, and all agreed that none of this could have been predicted. As we left the STU, Misti told me that it had felt funny to have these nurses hug her when she had never even seen them before in her life.

We talked about her stay at Suburban as we went back down the hospital's long halls and across the parking lot. As we passed the helicopter pad, I paused to tell her how the helicopter had landed with her at this very spot and how the nurses and doctors worked diligently to save her life. I explained to her that if this accident had to happen, it was best to have happened here rather than in a small town like Waynesboro, which had no STU. Though I did not say as much to Misti, I felt sure that without the specialized care she had gotten at Bethesda Suburban, she would probably not have made it.

Ten

After we left Suburban, we continued down Route 50 across Bay Bridge, finally turning down Coastal Highway and toward the bay. Having spent the previous four months away from anything really resembling home, I was excited to be going to Ocean City, which held so many happy memories for me. When we turned into the parking lot of our condo on Bayshore Drive, which backed onto the Chesapeake Bay, we were greeted by a sign that the other condo owners had hung over our porch: "Welcome, Misti." It was a kind gesture. I had been away from friends for a long time, and I was looking forward to reestablishing contact with people I'd known from before the accident.

But first we had to move ourselves in. Harry would be arriving the next day with more clothes and the comforts of daily life, but for now I had to get Misti and myself settled. It was immediately obvious that the small, two-bedroom condo had not been designed with wheelchairs in mind. I could maneuver Misti's chair up the small steps up to the front porch, but the doorway wasn't wide enough to accommodate the wheelchair. Though we would use the chair for walks and for transporting

Misti any real distance, we never brought it inside the house because it wouldn't fit through the doorways inside, nor would it fit into the bathroom or kitchen.

From the porch, I picked Misti up and carried her inside; she was still very thin, and though she'd put on a little of the weight she'd lost since the accident, I could carry her relatively easily. After a day on the road, Misti was content to watch TV while I unloaded the car, attached the handrails to the commode, and put away clothes. I fixed us a quick dinner and helped Misti eat, then decided to combine a trip to a nearby convenience store for milk and bread with a walk for Misti.

Later that night, we faced the first real challenge: showering Misti in the condo's small bathroom. This, it soon became clear, would have to be a multistep operation. I had to carry Misti in from the hall to the commode, set her down, and help her to undress. Then I had to lift her from the commode to the shower chair past the sliding shower doors—which only exposed half of the tub and shower and didn't provide much room to maneuver. After the shower, I had to reverse the process, step by step. Once Misti was showered and dressed and in bed, I returned to give the bathroom a thorough drying. I hoped I would get better at this quickly. A clean bathroom is a wonderful thing, but going through this every day would use up an awful lot of time and energy.

Harry arrived the next day, and when I showed him the problem with the shower, he said he'd install both an accordion door and a handheld shower head on a hose the next time he came down. That Sunday was Father's Day, and Misti gave her dad the woven door mat she had made for him in occupational therapy plus a card she had made on the computer before she left Bryn Mawr. Tears filled his eyes at Misti's loving efforts and then again when he had to leave us yet another time and make the long drive back to Waynesboro. While Misti and I continued to work on her various therapies in Ocean City, Harry would be working on the real estate development project back home that would, we hoped, pay the bills for the costly rehabilitation process.

The very next morning, Misti's therapies began again. Left to myself, I might have asked for a longer break between Misti's leaving Bryn Mawr and starting a full-fledged therapy schedule in Ocean City, but I also knew doing so might be dangerous. With any real kind of a break, Misti might regress and we'd just have to work harder to catch up.

From the first discussions about continuing Misti's rehabilitation in Ocean City, Cathy Cosgrove and the staff at Bryn Mawr had made it clear that routine would be important. We'd need to keep in mind that Misti would be starting over in a brand-new place—a highly stressful situation for someone in her condition—and just after a number of big, emotionally draining and possibly confusing events. With so much that was new, she could easily find herself swamped. Consistency was important, the professionals had stressed. We should avoid swapping time slots for the therapies; the changes would be easier for Misti to handle if she always had a particular therapy at a particular time on a regular schedule. Similarly, it would be best if Misti did not see much of Max until she'd really settled into a routine.

So, that first week was devoted to getting Misti acclimated. Monday, Anita Miller, a college student who would take care of Misti's cognitive retraining therapy, came by for a first session, and Cathy Payne, who would be Misti's physiotherapist, and her assistant, Laurie, came by to introduce themselves as well. Cognitive retraining was the only real therapy that first day, but over the course of the week, we added other therapies to the daily mix. One by one, Misti met all of the team, including Dave Delfanso, a kindly, thoroughly professional man, who would be the speech therapist, and Kim Chandler, the occupational therapist. By the end of the week, we'd been to the nursing home forty-five minutes away in Salisbury, where Cathy would run the physical therapy sessions. We'd also found the office of the doctor who would keep track of Misti's blood Tegretol level, and we met Dr. Carpenter, the psychiatrist we'd be consulting to help Misti and me deal with her emotional state and reactions to her dawning recognition of her deficits.

Overall, that first week in Ocean City went very well, and I felt very positive about the summer's potential. While nothing could replace the staff of Bryn Mawr, Cathy Cosgrove had clearly done a terrific job of putting together a good group of people to help with the therapies, and I was confident that Misti would continue her recovery in Ocean City.

Unfortunately, the calm and optimistic feeling of that first week didn't last. Though Misti generally cooperated with the therapists, it soon became clear that she considered the summer in Ocean City as vacation time, with fewer demands and rules than at Bryn Mawr. As a routine was established and therapies started to occupy most of her waking hours, Misti began to fight the schedule. She had not seemed to give much thought to Max the first week, when she hadn't seen him, but once he was allowed to visit, she was very upset that they weren't allowed to spend more time together.

According to the rules we'd all agreed to back in Malvern, Max could visit for half an hour three times a week and an hour on Saturdays. This would allow Misti time for therapies and the rest she needed after them. Things went fairly smoothly during the second week in Ocean City, but by the week after, both Misti and Max were trying to bend the rules. Max started stretching his visiting time to an hour or more every day. Since he didn't yet have a job, he had very little to do with his afternoons besides visiting Misti, and he often stayed through dinner and beyond. This put me in the position of traffic cop, enforcing the rules so that Misti could have a quiet evening and get her rest. When Max lingered through the early evening, and I said he had to leave, Misti would protest, saying that the movie or whatever they'd been watching on TV wasn't over yet. Eventually, we would only turn on half-hour shows or play videos that could be stopped at any point, but at the beginning of the summer, there were almost nightly quarrels over this issue, and Misti often ended up throwing full-scale tantrums.

Nor were Misti's evening tantrums always directed at me for making Max leave. Often, when Max finally said good-night, Misti would turn on him, accusing him of leaving to have sex with every girl in Ocean City. She told him that if he still found her desirable, he would do the same with her; and her accusations were always full of four-letter words. Though her ferocity sometimes scared him, for the most part, Max did his best to ignore Misti's accusations, certain they were a passing phase and that she'd soon be back to "normal." In any case, with Misti practically throwing herself at Max, I was thankful that we were in such confined quarters; it was easier for me to keep track of her every move. The last thing we needed at this point was a pregnancy.

Coping with Misti's therapy schedule and her emotional swings made for a very full day, and though I was spending a lot of time with the calendar, arranging, entering, and checking off therapists' and doctors' visits, I wasn't paying close attention to actual dates. One day, there was a knock at the door, and when I answered it a delivery man handed me a bouquet of flowers. As I opened the card, I realized that it was my wedding anniversary—June 25—and I'd completely forgotten. The card accompanying the flowers reminded me that after more than thirty years together, Harry still loved me. I didn't spend a lot of time berating myself for forgetting the date, because I knew I had my hands full just keeping Misti and me going, but I couldn't help feeling sad. One of the effects of Misti's accident had been to change our marriage from one of closeness and intimacy to a somewhat strained long-distance relationship. When I finished arranging the flowers on the dining room table, I sat down with the card in my hand and wondered with exhaustion whether Harry and I would every get that special closeness back.

⊚

Though Misti had made great progress at Bryn Mawr at the start of the summer, she was clearly still a patient recovering from brain trauma and coma. Her speech was slurred, and understanding her took some effort. Her vision was not good; even with glasses, she wasn't seeing very well. This affected her balance and made her cognitive retraining therapy, some of which depended on being able to see well enough to match shapes or read words, difficult. Her leg muscles were weak and needed to be built back up through exercise, and she still had weakness on her left side, including some paralysis on the left side of her face. Her memory, both short- and long-term, had been affected by the accident, and her ability to reason was faulty. In addition, her emotional state was volatile: Sometimes she was loving and sweet, but she was also moody, and she had tantrums when she was upset or frustrated.

The ultimate goal, of course, was to help Misti recover as much as possible in a pleasant setting that would allow her to accept that she had been badly injured and that serious problems remained without becoming so discouraged that she gave up. It was a tall order, but none of us was willing to give up now.

One afternoon shortly after we arrived in Ocean City, I got proof that Misti remembered the wild night at Bryn Mawr when I'd seen her reflection in the mirror. After lunch, I took her out in the wheelchair for a walk. As I pushed the chair over the uneven pavement and then down off the curb, Misti got impatient and loudly reprimanded me for my careless driving, threatening to replace me with someone who could do a better job. "I'm going to make you lose your driver's license," she threatened. But after only a few choice cuss words, she stopped long enough for me to interrupt her with, "Aw, don't give up on me now." Suddenly her head turned around much farther than I believed possible, and a small smile crossed her face as she replied, "Not now." The easy way the words came out and the teasing tone in her voice let me know that she, too, remembered the night the light shone in the mirror and she appeared to beg me not to give up on her.

Well, I hadn't then, and I wasn't about to now.

⊚

Early in July, Joan and Jerry Snyder dropped by for a visit. The Snyders had been of great help when Harry and I first decided to buy a place in Ocean City years before, and they were quite fond of Misti, who was about the same age as their two daughters. It was great to see these old friends, and when they left after a wonderful catch-up session, I started to get Misti ready for bed. Suddenly, she became violent, screaming four-letter words and throwing everything within reach. In the grips of some kind of emotional storm, she had absolutely no respect for anything and almost seemed to enjoy breaking the things that she thought I held dear.

I outweighed Misti by fifty pounds, but her fury gave her a terrifying strength. Any time I got close enough to try to calm her down and stop the destruction, she bit at me until I had to back away. Finally, I gave up, retreated to the other room, and waited until she fell asleep from sheer fatigue. She remained restless the entire night, and I, too, was restless, exhausted, and scared. This storm had seemed to come out of a clear blue sky, completely without warning.

When I sat down to think about this later, however, I realized that Misti was probably terribly tired and literally mind-boggled. She'd had three wild weeks, during which she'd left Bryn Mawr, gone home to Waynesboro and then on to Mercersburg for commencement, and then back to Bryn Mawr for a good-bye to the staff there. She'd then visited the STU at Suburban on the way down here to Ocean City, where she'd spent two full weeks meeting new therapists and doctors and getting used to the condo. After months of relative sameness, everything had changed at once. On top of this, she'd been visited by friends she hadn't seen in months and might not even have remembered. Her injured brain had probably overloaded and short-circuited as it tried to cope with all the changes at the same time. This very logical explanation for Misti's tantrum, however, did nothing to counteract the terror I'd felt at its suddenness and intensity. I'd never seen anything like it.

And as would often be the case when this kind of thing happened,

Misti was in poor shape the next day. Ordinarily, she required about twelve hours of sleep a day to rest and allow her brain to heal after a day of intensive therapy, but after an emotional storm like the previous night's, she needed even more rest. When Kim came for occupational therapy the next morning, Misti was in her own world, and therapy for the entire day was nearly useless.

This first emotional storm at Ocean City was the harbinger of a summer of emotional squalls and hurricanes. Some of them had to do with Misti's exhaustion and frustration: She was often very tired and wanted to stay in bed rather than get up for therapy, and she was frustrated at not seeing more of Max. And some of them, surely, had to do with her tangled emotional wiring. Somewhere inside, she had to be sad about what had happened to her. In addition, she was definitely tired of therapy and having to see me every waking hour of every day. Maybe, I thought, if she could cry to express her sadness at missing her friends or her frustration at having to be to be so dependent on me, her anger would be less; but with her emotions scrambled, anger seemed to be her only outlet. Sometimes I could tell that Misti was getting upset, but more often the devastating storms came out of nowhere. In fact, as the summer went on, they often occurred early in the day, when nothing particularly frustrating had yet happened. It was as if her brain was short-circuiting intermittently, and when that happened, there was hell to pay.

I got most of Misti's abuse, but I was not the only target. Everyone who worked with her became familiar with her storms and foul language, and for the most part, they just proceeded quite professionally to do their work. Usually, if no one got too upset or paid her outbursts too much attention, Misti would calm down relatively quickly.

As for myself, I'd seen and heard patients at Bryn Mawr persevere in bad language for quite some time, and I knew that this was a stage in Misti's recovery. However, the hurricane force of her rage was frightening. Sometimes, after she had finally dropped into sleep, I would look at her lovely and innocent face and marvel in utter disbelief at the vulgarity that poured from her mouth all day long. Some days were worse than others, but few days that summer were free from Misti's angry, aggressive behavior.

I noticed that she was usually less agitated when the therapists were around, though her reactions differed person by person. Misti had bonded well with most of the therapists—especially Laurie, Cathy

Payne's assistant—though that didn't save her from the outbursts. She sounded off at Anita more than the others, and she had more control when Lori and Kim were on site. Misti behaved best with Dave Delfanso, her speech therapist, perhaps because he represented more of an authority figure to her than the young women. Even so, she made it quite clear from the start that she didn't like him. Misti's general attitude toward people had changed since the accident. As she recovered, she had become very opinionated about the people she met. She either liked someone or she didn't; there was no middle ground. And she could be quite tactless in expressing herself. One day, after their speech therapy session had finished and Dave Delfanso had closed the door of the condo behind him, she yelled in her strongest voice, "He is queer, Mom. You know he is queer." Immediately, I said, "Please do not use the word 'queer.' A nicer word is 'gay,'" and then explained that he had a wife and twin daughters, which was hardly likely to be the case if he were gay. Her response was to glare at me with hatred and rage, saying "Go f—-yourself, bitch." The cuss word barely registered; in a shockingly short period of time, I had become accustomed to hearing Misti say four-letter words.

As at Bryn Mawr, an essential piece of life in Ocean City was the team meeting. I would take Misti up to Bryn Mawr for checkups several times over the course of the summer, and the doctors there were still directing the overall course of her rehabilitation, but the day-to-day strategy was decided at the general team meetings in Ocean City, which took place every two weeks. The meetings were attended by me and all the therapists, with Cathy Cosgrove driving down from Pennsylvania to chair them and act as liaison with the professionals at Bryn Mawr. The only team positions we were missing were those of physiatrist and psychiatrist: The Ocean City doctor who was checking Misti's Tegretol level was not a rehab specialist or an expert on brain trauma, and Dr. Carpenter was at his house on the shore only on weekends, when his regular practice in Baltimore was closed. So, we missed both the input and reassurance of a Dr. Audieh or a Dr. Armstrong, who could explain that Misti's upsetting behavior was typical of a patient recovering from traumatic brain injury and coma. I knew that Dr. Carpenter talked to Cathy Cosgrove, who passed along reports to Bryn Mawr, but it wasn't the same as having a knowledgeable rehab psychiatrist on call. And Dr. Carpenter had frustratingly little to say about the emotional storms that were plaguing our lives.

Perhaps because I was feeling so isolated—other than Misti and the therapists and doctors, I had time to see very few other people, particularly at the start of the summer—I always felt a load being lifted off my shoulders when I saw Cathy Cosgrove's car pull into our parking lot. Cathy was always very supportive. She was aware that the move from Bryn Mawr to Ocean City was likely to be difficult for both Misti and me, and she had called me every day the first week. She also told me that I could call her anytime; she even gave me her home number. As the summer went on, our twice-weekly conversations were immensely reassuring for me, especially when she offered to take on the role of the heavy in my fights with Misti about Max's visiting times.

On the first team meeting day, however, these patterns weren't yet established, and Misti considered Cathy her savior. Cathy barely got through the door before Misti launched herself at her, telling her that the rules about Max visiting were unfair, that she wasn't able to see him often enough. She demanded more freedom, including permission to go out with Max in his car and more time without me around. But Cathy, having anticipated this moment back at Bryn Mawr, was ready. She took charge immediately and issued a stern ultimatum: If Misti and Max could not follow the rules that had already been set up, as they'd both agreed back in Pennsylvania, and if Misti could not stand to live with me twenty-four hours a day, the only alternative was for her to go back into the Rehab at Bryn Mawr or some other kind of institutional living situation where she would not be allowed to see either Max or me on a regular basis.

Cathy's willingness to be the heavy took a lot of pressure off me, and Misti, chastened, promised to try harder to keep to the rules. From this point on, she agreed, Max would only be able to visit for an hour at a time during the work week and only when the visit was approved by me. On weekends, he would be able to visit for longer periods, unless she threw tantrums. I prayed the scheme would work this time.

Cathy then went one step further and decided to add a facilitator to our minirehab staff. It wasn't essential that the facilitator—a young person who could stay with Misti and keep her company while giving me some respite—be specially trained; what was important was that she get along well with Misti and be a companion, almost a friend. Since

Misti couldn't be left alone because of the threat of seizures, I'd had to be with her every hour of every day. The facilitator could step in to relieve me so I could do the grocery shopping, take a walk, go to church, or even take in a movie; she could also approve extra visits from Max if Misti had been behaving herself well. This might be a very good idea, I thought. Misti and I had been living in each other's pockets since arriving in Ocean City. Perhaps she would be less agitated if we were not together all of the time. The insurance company had already agreed to the arrangements, so adding another person would not be a problem financially.

Cathy then left after a private meeting with Misti where she emphasized, once again, that if things did not get better soon, she would have to make arrangements to have her admitted to an institution. Misti took this threat quite seriously and tried hard to improve her behavior.

July 4th fell on a Monday that year, and since therapists had the holiday off, it made a break in the schedule for Misti. Harry stayed for Saturday and Sunday, and Misti behaved herself well, with no tantrums. As always, Harry hated to leave, and we hated to see him go. It was harder to say good-bye at Ocean City than it had been in Paoli; the condo was a family place, where we'd always been happy together, and Harry having to leave us behind under these difficult circumstances seemed wrong.

On Monday, the traffic on Coastal Highway was horrendous, so we didn't want to drive anywhere. To fill an otherwise empty day, I took Misti for a long walk, and about a block from the condo, I helped her get up and had her push the empty wheelchair for a few feet. With great effort she succeeded and was as proud of herself as I was of her.

Later in the evening, Cathy Payne, the physical therapist, called to tell me about a new arrangement that would give me more free time. Twice a week, I would take Misti to Salisbury and drop her off at the gym in the nursing home; Dave Delfanso, the speech therapist, would pick her up and bring her back to Ocean City for her speech therapy session. This would not only give them more time together to work on her therapy in a casual, unstructured, and unpressured environment, but would also give Misti and me almost two additional hours break from one another's company every week. I thought she would like this idea a lot; even though she disliked Mr. Delfanso, she did like being out in the car, and especially being out in the car without me.

Arriving back at the condo after a visit to Dr. Carpenter the next Friday, Misti and I were thrilled to see Cork and Emily, who had come down to spend the weekend, bringing along Nickii, one of Misti's cousins. Nickii and Misti had been friends since childhood. Because the girls were the same age, Harry and I often brought Nickii with us on vacation as company for Misti, and Nickii's parents, Tom and Joyce, did the same. Now, Nickii would stay with us until Tom and Joyce came down to the shore for their vacation a week later.

Sunday evening, Max, Nickii, and a friend of Max's decided to take Misti for a walk. Max pushed Misti in the wheelchair and the others walked along side. As they headed off into the light of the early evening, the four of them made a pretty picture. However, I soon got a frantic call from Max telling me that Misti was throwing a major tantrum on the boardwalk. He and Nickii were both terrified, and I had to go get Misti, cutting through the crowd of curious and avid onlookers that had gathered. When I arrived, she and Max were arguing violently. Nickii and Max both told me that Misti had "lost it"—screaming, shouting accusations, hitting out wildly, and actually striking Nickii— but they weren't sure why. The tantrum had begun with Misti screaming that she did not want Nickii to stay with us, but it escalated into a real fight when Max offered to let Nickii stay at his place instead.

It was the first of a series of scenes we'd see again and again during the summer, with Misti accusing Max of being unfaithful to her. Now Misti accused him of wanting Nickii to stay with him so they could have sex. It took me hours to get her calmed down once I got her back to the condo. It seemed that we had made no progress on this front. Misti was putting two and two together and getting 112, and she was suspicious of nearly everyone and everything, especially when it came to Max. She was not jealous of her own girlfriends, such as Rani, but, when someone new came on the scene, even her cousin, she seemed to feel suddenly very inferior and became extremely possessive and accusatory.

After a week of being around the extremely volatile Misti, Nickii was very glad to see Tom and Joyce when they arrived in Ocean City for their vacation. In fact, she confided to Joyce that, as much as she loved Misti, she had been scared of her at times. She had never realized what recovery from brain trauma might involve. When Nickii described Misti's recurrent tantrums, Joyce reached into her background as a kindergarten teacher and suggested that we try a reward system to help Misti's regulate her behavior. It worked with her students, she said; maybe it would help with Misti.

Using a water glass as a pattern, Joyce and I cut "coins" from pieces of different colored posterboard. The coins had to be very large because Misti's vision was so poor. The yellow ones represented fifteen minutes, the red ones ten minutes, the blue ones five minutes, and the very valuable white ones thirty minutes. We then proceeded to print up a chart of rules. Max was allowed to visit for a total of ten hours a week. Each Sunday evening, Misti would receive enough coins to allow for full visitation time. During the week, she would be rewarded with more coins if she was especially good. However, she could also lose coins for unacceptable behavior. The chart clearly stated that cuss words cost a blue coin, or five minutes. Temper tantrums would cost ten minutes to an hour, depending on how long they lasted. Hitting, kicking, or biting would cost fifteen minutes to thirty minutes, depending on the severity; throwing anything would cost a yellow coin, or fifteen minutes. We made a bank from a box with a slot in the top. The top came off easily, allowing Misti access to the coins to pay for the privilege of visits with Max. Our hope was that she would soon learn to judge the value of the privilege and modify her behavior accordingly.

When Misti was introduced to the new reward and penalty program, she smiled, very confident it was going to afford her long hours with Max. She asked if she could keep the coin bank in her bedroom beside her bed; my coins, we agreed, would be kept in a Tupperware container on the top of the refrigerator, which she couldn't reach. Misti told Max about the coin bank, and he, too, was enthusiastic about the system and promised to help her remember how she wanted to behave.

The new system started on Sunday. When Max was ready to leave, Misti "paid" me the coins she owed for his visit—and without throwing a tantrum, because she wanted to hold on to the precious coins she had left. After her bath one night later in the week, the two of us sat and watched the boats and lights reflected in the Bay. How peaceful it all felt, how wonderful.

Before going to bed, I thanked God for Joyce's great idea, which was beginning to bring calm to our lives, for the place here at the beach to conduct the therapies outside of an institution, and for Cathy Cosgrove for finding us good therapists. I even thanked God for the weather, which had been beautiful, with almost no rain and yet without excessive heat. The flowers on the porch that I had received for Mother's Day were blooming beautifully and had doubled in size. I had always dreamed of spending a complete summer in Ocean City, and now Misti was continuing her recovery in this peaceful and beautiful place. I realized once again that if we each sit quietly for a few moments and count our blessings, we will be amazed at how many we find we have. As usual, I also had something to ask God for. That night, it was that my doctor's checkup the next day would go well. The doctors up at Paoli had insisted that I have my heart checked again, and if anything were really wrong with my health now, it would be very unfortunate for Misti.

The rest of the week did go well. I got a clean bill of health from the doctor, checked out a pool at an Ocean City health club for Misti's continued physical therapy, and had visits from the Snyders, as well as Joyce and Tom. Misti did well in therapy and had visits from one of the Snyders' daughters and a friend. When Harry called, he was delighted to hear that the behavior modification program was working for Misti, and he also said he would be coming down shortly to stay for a week.

Unfortunately, this idyllic time came to an end the following Saturday evening, when the erratic nature of recovery from brain trauma reasserted itself. Max was due to stop by, and as Misti began to count the coins she had remaining in her bank, she found that she had only one yellow and one white one, and she was not due to get more until the next day. She and Max wanted to watch a video, but if he could only stay one hour and fifteen minutes, they would have to cut the evening short. She immediately became furious and threw the box and the coins at me, screaming four-letter words.

Tom and Joyce arrived while Misti's tantrum was in full swing, and for the first time they saw the tremendous force of her anger. Joyce commented that she had never witnessed anything like it outside of *The Exorcist*. She and Tom offered to give me a break by taking Misti out for a drive and put her, still thrashing, kicking, and screaming obscenities, in their car. Tom drove away, with Joyce and Misti using the back seat as their battleground.

Simultaneously relieved and worried, I walked back into the condo to try to clean up after Misti's tantrum. When I finished, I slumped into a chair, empty of all emotion. I felt like a dark shell of a person, without a living spirit. I completely lost track of the passing of time and was only jolted back to life when I heard the car pull up in the parking lot. I ran to the door and saw, from the familiar mess on Misti's clothes, that Tom and Joyce had taken her to TCBY. Misti was quiet, and Joyce looked as though she had lost the battle but won the war. She helped me bathe Misti and get her to bed. The tantrum had lasted several hours, and Misti was so tired that she fell asleep almost immediately.

We kept trying the coin system, using the coins to reinforce good behavior and offering as rewards computer games, trips to TCBY, or an extra video with Max, but after about a month, I had to concede defeat. The coin system and other reinforcers were a good idea, but they didn't work for Misti. Penalty and reward systems worked well with people who could reason consistently, and for now anyway, brain trauma made that impossible for Misti.

It was around this time that I began to feel uneasy about whether Dr. Carpenter was helping at all. Misti's emotional state was nearly as bad as it had been back before she had moved into the Laurels several months before. No one was able to predict how she would react to any situation. In spite of this, Dr. Carpenter never seemed to have much to say to me—no comments on Misti's relationship with Max or with me, or about her frequent angry and jealous outbursts. In fact, he never even asked me to clarify anything that Misti said, which was rather odd because her speech was still quite slurred and difficult to understand. When I mentioned the various forms of behavior modification we had tried with Misti, he had no suggestions to offer. And he never called anyone at Bryn Mawr directly to speak about Misti's case, leaving those discussions to Cathy Cosgrove. At first I thought Dr. Carpenter merely had his own style, and I tried to be patient, since all the other therapists that Cathy had found were working out so well. But the situation was clearly problematic, and it seemed to be getting worse.

Midway through July, Max's parents came down from their home in Gaithersburg, Maryland, to visit Max, and I prepared lunch for all of us. Though we all enjoyed a pleasant meal, it was clear that this wasn't purely a pleasure trip for the Greys. After lunch, his father came down hard on Max because after a month in Ocean City, he was neither employed nor actively seeking employment. Anthony sternly reminded him that though he and his mother were paying the rent for the condo, Max must now grow up and take some responsibility by getting a job. If he was not employed by the end of the week, Anthony said, he and Brenda would return to Ocean City to pick Max up and move him back to Gaithersburg.

Part of me hoped fervently that Max would not be able to find a job and have to go home. That way, we would avoid countless future arguments about how much time Misti and Max could spend together. Of course, this was just a pipe dream, because every fast food restaurant in town had "Help Wanted" signs in the windows. Ocean City is a haven for teens seeking summer work; the only problem is finding an affordable place to live. And Brenda and Anthony had already taken care of that problem for Max.

While the Greys visited with Misti—they were delighted to see her looking so much better—Max stormed out with an angry look on his face. He returned an hour later, employed. The very next day he would be starting at Burger King, just a few blocks up Coastal Highway. Though I'd have preferred that Max leave Ocean City, I took some relief from the fact that he had finally gotten a job. Surely Misti would have to recognize that if Max worked eight hours a day and slept eight hours, he would not have as much time to visit her.

But even this rag of comfort soon disappeared. Whether or not Misti could do the arithmetic of a twenty-four-hour day, she was very upset that Max wasn't as available to her. Furthermore, he worked the late night shift, and Misti was sure that he was taking the girls who worked with him back to his condo after work to party, and as she put it, "to f—." Max did his best to persuade her that this was not the case, but to little avail. Misti remained jealous and accusatory, and anyone could become the target of her wrath at a moment's notice.

In addition to the exhausting daily tantrums, I was worried because Misti was still not able to cry or to express sadness. When I mentioned this to Dr. Carpenter, he seemed to understand nothing about the effects of brain trauma, in spite of the conversations I knew he had been having with Cathy Cosgrove. I found myself becoming increasingly doubtful about his skills, and I told the team and ACT in mid-July that I felt he was an inappropriate choice to care for Misti.

The next weekend really put the cap on the situation. Misti and I had fought the summer traffic all the way up Coastal Highway for our regular 5:00 P.M. appointment, only to find that Dr. Carpenter was not there. We waited on the porch for an hour, both of us doing a slow burn. Finally, it was clear to me that he was not going to show up; later I learned that he was not coming down for this weekend and had neglected to call us and let us know. Misti was so angry and frustrated at this rude treatment that she threw a fit, and it took me over half an hour just to get her back into the car. Once inside she kicked and screamed the entire one hundred blocks back down Coastal Highway. By the time I got her calmed down and fed, it was time for bed. Had I been able to get anyone from ACT on the phone on Friday night at 9:00, they would have gotten an earful, but since this was not possible, I had to wait until Monday morning.

All weekend, I mulled over the situation, returning over and over to the same irrefutable points. We needed access to a full-time psychiatrist, not one who made himself available only during the occasional hour in order to be able to use his summer home in Ocean City as a tax write-off. How would Misti make progress without a good doctor who was familiar with the residual effects of brain trauma? Without the best of doctors, how would we get the best of results?

On and on my mind whirled, until I realized that one could find fault with anyone or anything if one tried hard enough. But the fact remained that I was fed up, and rightly so. In general, ACT had done a good job, but not all of their choices were bound to work out. I had changed since Misti's accident. No longer was I someone who would meekly accept whatever was offered. Now I was more aggressive, willing to go to any lengths to get what Misti needed.

At 9:00 A.M. on the following Monday, Cathy Cosgrove took a call from me that carried the full force of a seven-millimeter Magnum. As always, she calmed me down, assuring me she would find another psychiatrist for Misti. True to her word, she called back several days later with a referral to a new doctor. The new doctor, she explained, also only spent weekends in the Ocean City area, but she assured me that Dr. Williams was extremely well-qualified and would be able to handle the situation professionally. Time would tell.

The following Friday evening, we headed north on Coastal Highway to Fenwick Island and took Route 54 to our destination, a town house on one of the many canals. The door bell was answered by a very calm, gentle-looking man, who welcomed us inside a lovely house whose interior was evenly coated throughout with cat fur. The fur was the calling card of two Himalayan cats, one very mellow and always in plain sight, the other terrified at the sight of humans and only glimpsed skittering out of the room. The man with the gentle face was Dr. Williams, and though I was now wary of psychiatrists, I was also willing to give him a chance.

Eleven

One Friday night, late in July, Harry arrived in Ocean City very excited. They were finally about to break ground on his project in Waynesboro—Morningstar Heights, a development of fifteen town houses to be built on a tract of wooded land northeast of town. Morningstar Heights would be the first big project of his second career. It was something of a risk and certainly involved a lot of work, but it carried great potential for both profit and satisfaction. It was a point of pride that the area's best contractor would be working for him on the development. We spent the evening catching up on family matters and celebrating the beginning of Harry's new career.

As was his habit, Harry got up early the next morning and took a long bicycle ride around Ocean City to get his exercise. By the time he returned, the day was half over, and I was angry and hurt that he had not stepped in to take over with Misti and give me a little free time. I knew he had been very preoccupied with Morningstar Heights and that he needed some relaxation, but so did I. Despite our frequent phone conversations, I had the feeling that he thought I had spent the previous month on vacation, that he did not realize that the only time I actually got some sun was when I took Misti out for a walk in the wheelchair. Later, when Misti threw the inevitable tantrum, Harry made it clear he was annoyed, telling me the problem was that I was "picking on her." If I'd just let her do things in her own way, at her own pace, everything would be okay. He thought I should ease up, let the therapists and doctors handle Misti, and not try so hard to control everything. But my experience had been that most of the doctors and therapists had only minimal expectations of her and that it was up to the family to keep Misti's rehabilitation going. I also told him I thought we'd do better with more help from him when he was here. Needless to say, when he left he was angry with me for expecting too much of him.

That evening, Misti and I played several of the computer games provided by the CAT fund as part of her cognitive retraining, and Misti clearly enjoyed herself. When she began to show signs of getting tired, I suggested she go to her room and get her night clothing. At this, she lashed out defiantly, pushing the keyboard aside with a quick swing of her right hand and sending the computer mouse flying up against the wall. "How the f—-do you expect me to do that when I cannot even walk?" she screamed, as though it weren't part of her nightly routine to help get herself ready for bed. For some reason—maybe my anger at Harry or the frustrations built up over the last several months—I found myself swearing back. "The same f——ing way a dog carries its pups," I said, continuing with, "I am tired of your damn laziness. You expect me to wait on you hand and foot, and I am tired of it. Just who the hell do you think you are anyway?" Then I stopped and watched silently as she crawled down off the chair on the floor and slowly, on hands and knees, made her way to her room. When she neared the door, she lost her balance and fell over. Guilt clenched my heart like a vise as I heard the deafening crack of her head hitting the wall; for the first time in my life, I had said the f-word aloud and already I had been punished. I tried to pick her up and comfort her, but she started hitting, clawing, and biting. My left hand took the hardest bite and bright red blood ran down my thumb. When I pulled back my hand to look at it, I dropped my guard and felt her teeth sink into my breast, breaking the skin even through my clothes. But she was too tired to continue, so the battle ended with her threatening to kill me. Nonetheless, she let me tuck her into bed and fell asleep almost immediately.

By the time I had gotten ready for bed, I was almost too exhausted to sleep. I was also frightened, stunned by the raw physical power behind her fury. My night was very uncomfortable, and what little rest I managed was broken when a neighbor's disoriented cat came in through a door propped open to catch the breeze from the Bay. After I escorted the cat out, it was impossible to get back to sleep. Instead, I went back inside, put an ice pack on my breast, and tried to distract myself with a movie on TV.

As the summer's difficult weeks went on, I had to admit that Dr. Williams was an improvement on Dr. Carpenter. He was on time for appointments, he was gentle and calm, he was attentive to Misti and to my questions, and he was willing to listen when I told him about Misti's emotional difficulties. However, after a meeting with Harry and me, he said that he feared that the Morningstar family had become somewhat dysfunctional. On the basis of what we told him, Misti and I had become too enmeshed with one another and isolated from other people, while Harry was too far away and too removed from the day-to-day reality of Misti's and my life. Though he said it kindly, Dr. Williams said he found it difficult to believe that before February 5, 1988, we had been a close and caring family. He apparently didn't understand that an acci-

dent like Misti's could create the devastating situation we found ourselves in. Though we certainly had our share of problems, we were not
a family dealing with a child who had some lifelong mental problem or
a chemical imbalance; we were a family dealing with a child who had
suffered brain trauma.

At the same time, I had to admit that there was some truth to what
Dr. Williams had said. Although I had never really thought about it in
those terms before, I realized that I had somehow believed that a
tragedy like this should make members of a family love each other
more and pull them closer together, not the opposite. Well, here was the
test: Misti and I were alone in Ocean City, and the rest of our family
was over two hundred miles away.

All the questions I had refused to ask myself over the past lonely
months began to haunt me. What was Harry's life in Waynesboro like
without me? How was Harry handling the stress of starting a new business, of sleeping alone at night? How were Chuck and Cork explaining
the absence of Nana to their children? Did my friends realize there was
an empty chair at their meetings? Who was going out on the decorating
jobs when my clients called for assistance? And how was Mommie handling caring for Daddy without my help?

◎

Though our expenses in Ocean City were lower than they'd been up in
Malvern, money was still extremely tight. I didn't make many long-distance calls, even though I was very lonely, and most evenings after I'd
put Misti to bed I was too tired to do much more than jot an occasional
note in my diary or watch TV. And perhaps because they'd heard that
Misti and I were in Ocean City, almost everyone else—our friends and
even many of our relatives—seemed to assume we were at the shore
just to have fun and no longer needed the special kind of support they'd
offered in such abundance while Misti was in Bryn Mawr.

One exception was Joyce, who made a real point of staying in touch.
And we saw a good deal of the minister from the Lutheran church in
Ocean City, who had been making regular weekly home visits to us
since we'd arrived and had invited us both to attend church when Misti
was able. Once Cathy Cosgrove added the facilitator to the team, I was
able to go to church alone, but I looked forward to taking Misti along
with me.

At the suggestion of Kim, the occupational therapist, the facilitator accompanied Misti and me as we attended church one Sunday. We all listened to the sermon, planning to discuss it when we got home and to share our interpretations of what the minister had been telling the congregation. But from the beginning of our lunchtime discussion, it was evident that Misti was not retaining much in her short-term memory. And as we continued to talk, it was obvious that she did not understand what little she had been able to retain; it was also clear that the most outstanding thing on her mind was the time Max would arrive for a visit. Max's presence at Ocean City was certainly proving distracting: When we succeeded in getting Misti's mind focused on anything else, we seemed to make some progress, but getting her to focus on anything or anyone other than Max was a huge chore.

At the same time, Misti had begun to understand that she had deficits remaining from the accident. We saw this one day when Anita decided that as part of the cognitive retraining therapy, she and Misti would go to the movies. The plan was that during the movie Anita would point out certain things to Misti and later they would see how much she could remember. Their first foray was to see an early show of *Big*, and though Anita reported that Misti enjoyed the movie, when they talked about it later, Misti was unable to remember what it had been about. Though no one was blaming her for the memory lapse, she apparently felt we were, and she flew into a rage and would not be comforted.

Misti was trying very hard, and we were careful to reinforce this, always praising her for her hard work. We pointed out every little bit of progress, and even when she could not do what she was asked, we always told her we knew how hard she was trying. But brain trauma has a harsh way of changing not only the life of the person affected, but that of everyone around her. For instance, before the accident, Misti had always been able to work out conflicts reasonably well. Though she was an intense and dramatic person, she had always been able to calm down and see reason. Well, Misti was the still an intense and dramatic person, but now she had significant memory and emotional problems. It was as though she could not modulate her emotional response to any situation. Her emotions were turned on loud, and it was very hard for her to adjust the volume.

Misti could present her case about a problem most emphatically, discuss the situation with me or Cathy Cosgrove, and even come to an acceptable solution. But then she would forget all about the conversation and the agreement shortly afterward. Some nights I wondered if she had actually fallen asleep or had just passed out from sheer exhaustion after all of the day's conflicts. Most of Misti's dramas that summer were about seeing Max, and Cathy Cosgrove was often called in to arbitrate. Cathy had had a lot of experience with similar situations, and she wasn't impressed with Misti's dramatic presentations. However, that didn't mean she had any better luck getting her to stick to agreements than I did because Misti just plain didn't remember from one day to the next what she'd agreed to. Because she couldn't remember, it was hard for us to have a sense that we were moving forward.

Nor was it easy for anyone to get Misti to change her mind once she made it up or to shake her from an idea, however faulty. For instance, when we went to the nursing home in Salisbury for physical therapy twice a week, Misti always said hello to a dapper elderly gentleman who sat inside the door of the nursing home in his wheelchair. As I pushed Misti's chair past him, he would smile and say, "Good morning, bright sunshine," and she did her best to acknowledge him and looked forward to seeing him. After one visit, however, we learned that he had passed away, and this realization was very hard on Misti. She began to complain that seeing the old people at the nursing home depressed her, though she didn't mind the physical therapy. She said that seeing the elderly residents reminded her that she had become "an old cripple long before her time," and she began equating her condition with being close to death. Nothing I could say—not that she was very young, or that she was getting better, not worse—would shake her from this notion. Days like this were very hard indeed, and I found myself saying often, "Thank you, God, for getting me through one more day, and let tomorrow be better, please."

Therapies continued, and Misti made slow but steady progress on a number of fronts. Despite her apparent hostility toward him, Dave Delfanso was devoted to her and very patient. The condo was so small that I could not help hearing the two of them when they were working in speech therapy. At the beginning of the summer, Misti's speech was more garbled than it had been when she had just started to talk as a toddler, and the only time it was clear was when she used profanity. Once more I wondered whether the experts had been right in saying that she could not get better. Though Dave repeatedly urged her to sing—a standard technique used by speech therapists to help strengthen the voice and add expression—Misti adamantly refused. After an initial trial, she wouldn't let Dave make a recording of her voice, either. When she listened to the first audiotape, she began to recognize that she had real problems in speaking. I suspect that until she actually heard the tape, she had been able to persuade herself that the problems were minor or the result of other people not listening well or paying close enough attention. She didn't want to accept the fact that she couldn't speak even recognizably, and she objected to the videotaping as well.

Dave was the first therapist to offer Misti a real challenge. Most of the other therapists didn't push her very hard to do things she didn't want to do. She didn't react well to his pushing and was often uncooperative. But he was creative as well as soft-spoken, and however hostile Misti might be, he continued to work with her, giving her encouragement every step of the way. Though she still signed when she was very tired and speech was just too much of an effort, the hard work of speech therapy and daily mouth and tongue exercises began to pay off. Her speech slowly improved and became clearer. An added bonus to her working with Dave was the fact that he was happy to incorporate Misti into his family to help, and she got along famously with his sixteen-year-old twin daughters.

Misti tried doing some physical therapy in the pool in Ocean City as she had at Bryn Mawr, but the water was too cold and the therapists were afraid the temperature would damage her muscles. At the condo, we tried to get her to crawl as much as possible to improve her balance and strength as a preliminary to walking. At the beginning of the summer, she would get up on all fours only to fall over on one side because her balance was so poor. We always cheered her on and praised her efforts so that she was never embarrassed to be crawling, but the clear memory of how much better she had done at only five months broke my heart a little each day. Still, exercise and therapy were strengthening her muscles, and the effort she put into crawling was improving her balance. By the middle of the summer, she had improved markedly, and she was able to get around the condo with amazing speed, moving quickly from room to room and even answering the door when the therapists knocked. When Ora and Goldie came down for a day trip in July, Misti was excited to show them that she could now get out of bed by herself and stand up in the kitchen by holding onto the cabinets.

One of the therapies Misti most enjoyed was cooking. This had never been one of her major interests before the accident, but she had done some cooking at the Rehab and she continued to do so in Ocean City. We would read through a recipe, measure the ingredients, and line them up on the counter so there was never a question as to whether we had added them or not. She especially liked making peanut butter pie for the team meetings and was very proud when I explained to guests that she had made something they were eating.

Whenever possible, we tried to combine therapies, both for efficiency and to keep Misti from getting bored. One of these combined practical therapies was having her help with the grocery shopping, which offered a combination of physical, occupational, and cognitive therapies. Misti helped make up the grocery lists, which required thinking about what we needed, and she got to practice walking by pushing the cart in the store. The therapist held on to the front of the shopping cart so it wouldn't run out of control, and Misti used the cart itself like a walker. She was thrilled to be doing this, feeling that she looked just like the other people in the store and not like a crippled person. Furthermore, most of the other customers at the grocery store were older people and less likely to stare or make embarrassing remarks.

Whenever Misti was doing well by making an effort to control her emotions, sticking with cognitive therapy even when it was tedious, or cooperating with Dave Delfanso even though she hated the sound of her own voice, we did what we could to reward her. Although money was tight, after a good week we would stop for a milkshake at a local spot on the way back from Dr. Williams's on Friday night. We also went out for breakfast most Monday mornings, when the crowds of vacationers thinned out. We usually went to Phillips by the Sea, a restaurant that was run by a young man who had become wheelchair bound after an accident. The staff there was always sympathetic to Misti without being condescending, and they made an appreciative fuss over her.

Even though Misti was making progress, there were days when she seemed to slide backwards, when therapy seemed almost futile. At times like that, the idea of going on seemed beyond me. To keep my spirits up, I would watch a few of the videos we had made of Misti at Bryn Mawr, so I could appreciate how far she had already come. And I always tried to think of the people who were worse off—my parents, for instance, or some of the people I remembered from the Rehab. Remembering them, I tried to give thanks for what we had and to stop lamenting the loss of the life we had had before.

Sometimes, however, this did not work. Sitting alone one evening, after an especially hard day, I found myself thinking the unthinkable: Might it have been better if Misti had died? The loss would have been devastating, but after a period of mourning, the beautiful memories of our vivacious daughter would linger intact, always with the certainty that she would have found the cure for Alzheimer's disease or AIDS as she had hoped. Although we would wonder if she would someday have married and blessed us with grandchildren, the lovely memories of her childhood and youth would have carried us to the end of our lives. Misti would have remained forever perfect in our minds, not difficult or wearing or incomprehensible as she was so often now.

I was instantly ashamed of my thoughts, but the reality was that she would never become a doctor, never have a chance to make that dream a reality, and I winced as I contemplated what the world had lost. With all the conviction of motherhood, I *know* that Misti would have made a difference, that she would have contributed greatly in the world of scientific research. Once she had matter-of-factly pulled down As in difficult subjects, securely on track for college and then medical school. Now, she was having to work terribly hard each day just to do the simplest things.

In August, therapies went on as\ usual, but with an added bonus. Harry came down to stay for a full week. It promised to be a great time, a pleasant return to regular family life. Harry would take Misti to her therapies in Salisbury, and we would take in a movie one evening. We would take Max along for dinner, and the four of us would go for walks on the boardwalk.

According to Dr. Williams, this week of family life should put Misti on the road to recovery. With a present and fully functional family, everything would be wonderful. Not! Somehow, whenever Misti threw a tantrum, it was still my fault. First Harry and then the doctor told me that I was at fault for the way I treated Misti. Now, exhausted and recognizing that the situation was indeed very bad, I could only think their accusations were right. I was picking on her, said Harry, so I backed off, watching him handle Misti the "proper way." Under his supervision, however, Misti's behavior was the same, the only difference being that with Harry on the premises I could actually go to sleep when I went to bed at night.

Unfortunately, Harry did not fare as well. He never slept well the first night in any house, and his sleep was broken two nights in a row by lost resort visitors knocking drunkenly at the door and by Misti's restlessness. Lack of sleep and concern about his project back in Waynesboro put Harry on edge, as did his frustration over not quite knowing how to help Misti.

Still, it was great to have Harry around, and we did in fact all go out for dinner one night and took a nice walk on the boardwalk. However, Misti also sensed her father's tension without quite understanding it. As always, things she did not understand tended to irritate her, affecting her mood. Harry was sure that if he just got strict with her and gave her firm commands, she would behave as well as she had before the accident, but this treatment only aggravated the situation, and the emotional storms began. Soon Harry and Misti were nearly at each other's throats, and Harry stormed out—but not before telling me that this was all my fault because I did not discipline her.

I dropped into a chair in fatigue and tried once again to sort things out. First, I had been blamed for being too strict, for picking on Misti. Now the problem was that I was not being assertive enough. Could it be true that it was all my fault, that I was a failure as a mother, caretaker, wife, and perhaps even as a human being? Maybe I had never been a success at anything, maybe everyone who came in contact with me had been pulled down because of me.

Shortly thereafter, Harry returned to Waynesboro, and I was once again in sole charge of Misti. There was no time for self-pity; time continued to speed by with daily therapies, daily tantrums, occasional visits from friends, and of course we had to keep up with the visits to Dr. Williams and to the other doctor for blood tests of the Tegretol level in Misti's body. This last precaution was an irritating chore, since it involved fighting traffic in Ocean City, but the Bryn Mawr team had made it clear that the drug was necessary to control possible seizure activity.

Determined to get more information, I took advantage of the services of the facilitator and spent some time at the local library. In reading some medical books there, I learned that, though Tegretol was preventing Misti from having grand mal (full-body) seizures, it was unlikely to have any effect on different types of seizures, outbursts the book called "emotional seizures." This information lit a bright bulb in my head, and when we returned to Bryn Mawr a bit later for a checkup,

I questioned the doctors there. Yes, they told me, Misti's tantrums could be related to seizure activity; they could also be due to brain malfunction.

One of the doctors there used his hands in an attempt to show me what was happening in Misti's brain. Lining up his hands horizontally, finger tip to finger tip, with palms facing, he explained that his fingers represented properly functioning brain circuits, with nerve impulses jumping in an orderly fashion from thumb to thumb, index finger to index finger, and so on. But Misti's brain had been injured, and so the circuits no longer lined up properly. Instead, impulses were jumping in a disorganized way from ring finger to index finger, from thumb to little finger. There was nothing, he stressed, that I or anyone else could do to prevent her brain from misfiring right now. Nothing I was doing could be contributing to the problem, either. Misti's outbursts were purely a matter of brain injury.

When I heard this news, I felt extraordinary relief. Misti's outbursts were not all my fault, contrary to the psychiatrist's speculations and Harry's accusations. I had been feeling guilty unnecessarily. In fact, if this had been explained to me before we left the Rehab, I would have been confident all along that I was doing the correct thing. But I hadn't known the proper questions to ask, and the doctors had not volunteered this explanation before, so we had all suffered. What was done was done, but as I drove back down to Ocean City, I had a lot of time to consider how much easier the summer might have been if I had known more about brain trauma.

○

As August wore on, the need to see more of the family began to eat away at me. After months on my own, I felt hollow, with an emptiness that even the best of memories could not fill. Though I often told Misti about our family life back in Waynesboro, trying to bridge the gaps in her memory, those memories of happier times seemed to be from another life.

One night, my reveries on the subject were interrupted by the ringing phone. It was Cathy Cosgrove. Was she psychic or just sensitive to my feelings of emptiness? In any case, she suggested that we bring my mother down to Ocean City for a visit. I tried explaining to her that this would be next to impossible, since my mother's eight-day-a-week job as Daddy's caretaker made even a phone call a major task. Even with a full-time nurse in the house to help, an Alzheimer's patient is not easy to care for. At my parents' house, the living room furniture had been put in storage, and a hospital bed and wall unit for the necessities of my father's care now filled the room; a Hoyer lift, to turn him in bed, stood in a corner. My mother, whose own health was fragile due to polio in childhood and diabetes as an adult, had had to become familiar with adult diapers, bed sores, male external catheters, and total hygiene care for another human being. In the ordinary course of life, one seldom considers such things as how difficult brushing the teeth of an unwilling person can be. Now, my mother was taking care of these things in Waynesboro, while I was doing the equivalent in Ocean City.

However, with the help of the Aetna nurse on our case, Cathy arranged for Mommie to come down by bus and visit for a week, while my father was cared for at a local nursing home. A facilitator came in to take care of Misti while I made the twenty-block trip to the bus station to pick Mommie up. I knew that it was hard for her to take off on her own for the first time in fifty years. Before my father's illness, she had always been taken care of, first by her parents and siblings, and then by my father, a kind and gentle man. But once Daddy was diagnosed with Alzheimer's she had become strong, taking on the endless, trying task of caring for him.

Actually, their lives had never been all that easy. Besides raising me and my brother, they took intermittent care of two of my cousins, tending to them as if they were their own. They were sorely tried when my handsome, winsome, and daredevilish cousin Jim quit school and ran off to join the Navy, lying about his age. With the help and intervention of my father, Jim was allowed to stay in the service, eventually becoming a pilot flying secret missions for the government. Then, one day Jim's plane crashed spectacularly, leaving him with crushed legs, a broken back and neck, and fractures in both arms. He died two days later, still flirting with the nurses, leaving the family broken-hearted.

Remembering past tragedies, I was determined to enjoy my mother's visit and to see to it that she enjoyed it as well. Mommie was delighted to see Misti's progress, though she couldn't help crying at the sight of her granddaughter crawling on all fours, and she was stunned at the ferocity of her tantrums. The week flew by, and too soon she had to board the bus for her return trip and to face the ambulance bringing Daddy back to the house. But it had been good to see her, and she had certainly become aware that day-to-day life was not easy for Misti and me, even if we were at the beach.

❂

Though the therapies and doctors' appointments provided a steady routine, each week took on its own flavor depending on errands we had to run and who might be visiting. For instance, one day, after a lot of preparation and persuasion, we took Misti to the dentist to have cement from her old retainer removed from her teeth. One day in August, we celebrated her birthday. Three times over the course of the summer, we made the trip up to Bryn Mawr so that the rehabilitation specialists there could monitor Misti's progress.

In any given week, friends from Waynesboro or Mercersburg might drop by for a few minutes to chat, or Chuck or Cork, whose flexible work schedules allowed them time to drop in for a weekday afternoon now and again. Misti also had a few letters and phone calls from Odette. But it tended to be a feast or famine situation, and if company for Misti arrived during therapy, they had to wait until the session was over.

The visitors who came least often tended to be upset at seeing Misti's slow recovery, and, though most of them handled it well, it was clear that they felt helpless when they couldn't understand something Misti was saying or doing. Those who visited more often could see the progress she was making and were able to be encouraging and to try to engage her in conversation. Rani was a particularly loyal visitor and came down several times over the summer. She was always happy to accommodate herself to whatever was going on and whoever else might be there, even accompanying us up to Bryn Mawr for one of Misti's checkups there. It was great to see these visitors, for both Misti and me, because they provided us with a link to the world that didn't involve therapy and reminded us of just why we were doing all the rehab work. Further, they brought me into touch with people I wasn't necessarily responsible for and helped ease my isolation.

The idea of the facilitator giving me a break to see friends was wonderful, but in fact, I usually spent the free time doing housework or grocery shopping rather than resting or getting together with friends. I did get to see one movie, and I tried to call my mother once a week, but I didn't have time to do much reading or even letter writing, though I was always glad to get mail.

Harry tried to get down to Ocean City as often as possible, but he was usually able to manage only a day here and there. We both hated that he had to leave at the end of a visit, but he had a hard time seeing Misti go through the difficulties of rehabilitation, and taking care of his responsibilities in Waynesboro was a way for him to help. When I told him about the Bryn Mawr doctor's explanation for Misti's tantrums, Harry took it in without saying much. But later in the month, he came down for the weekend and announced that the two of us were getting away on our own. He'd arranged to have a facilitator stay with Misti for a few days and took me off to a lovely hotel. It was good to be away, though I can't claim I was very scintillating company. In fact, I was so relieved at not having to be on call twenty-four hours a day that I spent a lot of the weekend just sleeping.

As the summer wound to a close, I was almost spent. As exhausted as I was, however, I knew that the time in Ocean City was serving its purpose. Misti was slowly but surely making progress. And as time went on, she seemed to become happier. I loved watching her smile, and the longer therapy went on, the more the left side of her mouth seemed to respond. The paralysis was not nearly as bad as it had been a few months before. By the end of August, there was a lovely gleam in her eyes at the anticipation of doing something she had been promised, whether going to the movies with her facilitator, spending a Saturday with Dave Delfanso's daughters at the Salisbury zoo, or spending an evening with her physical therapist Laurie and her husband at a concert.

Still, it was by no means smooth sailing, even in August. Brain trauma remained brain trauma, which is to say, unpredictable. Though the situation with Max became a little easier when his schedule required him to work evenings and we no longer had nightly fights about his visits, Misti continued to make all sorts of accusations about his morals and conduct. Max remained remarkably loyal, and when he could, he went along with us for visits to the doctor and psychiatrist. But he became moodier as the summer went on, which in turn had its effect on Misti. Not for the first time, I wondered if Max felt trapped— by a job he hated and a girlfriend who had been brain injured and wasn't recovering very quickly. This certainly was not the way he would have planned to spend the summer.

One Friday evening toward the end of the summer, as we were driving up the Coastal Highway to Dr. Williams's, Misti started screaming, then opened the car door and tried to jump out. Fortunately, her shoulder harness held her in and the force of the rushing air pushed the door back in and closed it. Usually, Misti liked going to see Dr. Williams—she liked him, she liked going to his house, and above all, she liked seeing his cats. She often made a game of guessing where they'd be when we arrived. This evening, though, Misti was clearly unhappy. While she continued to scream, I fought the traffic to get off the highway. Finally, I was able to turn onto a side street and stop, where I did my best to soothe her. Knowing that I must hold my emotions in check, I kept control, then got us back on the highway, turning in the direction of the much-needed psychiatrist.

Unfortunately, the only comfort there came from the two cats, as Dr. Williams told me yet again that Misti's continuing emotional problems arose from my overconcern with her and from the failings of our dysfunctional family. At this, the familiar, near-incapacitating guilt descended, nearly choking the breath from my body. But then I recalled that however kind and well-intentioned, Dr. Williams was not an expert on the cruelties of brain trauma and that he probably didn't know what was really happening with Misti day to day. How could his "reading up" on the subject begin to explain how we had been living since the spring? He was not dealing with it twenty-four hours a day as I was. On the days he gave me advice for dealing with Misti, he probably got a good night's rest, had time for exercise and regular meals, and in general was able to live a decent life. Maybe I could be handling things better, but the truth was our family life had altered in a big way with Misti's accident and would be altered perhaps for the rest of our lives. Tonight, while Dr. Williams went out for a pleasant dinner or sat watching TV with his cats in his lap, I would be tending once again to Misti and her unpredictable emotional reactions to life. I wondered how well he would do after months and months of this.

After dinner that evening, the tantrum forgotten, Misti and I sat on the dock, and she brought up the subject of ballet. She had remembered that she was once an accomplished ballerina and she asked if I thought she would ever dance again. This was a hard subject to discuss, and I told her that we could not dwell on what we used to be able to do. If I did that, I said, I would cry every day over many things. I explained that as we get older we are all unable to do things we did in our younger years. She replied, "I grew old very quickly, didn't I?" Though she was no longer equating getting older with dying, her question was still poignant, and there was no answer I could make.

⑨

As Misti continued to recover, life became a bit more normal. Not surprisingly, given that we were in an oceanside resort, she sometimes wanted to sunbathe. I let her do so, but cautiously, having learned a lot since the first time she'd gone sunbathing back in June. She had quickly gotten a bad burn because the medication for controlling seizures had made her very sensitive to the sun. A neighbor's suggestions of cold tea compresses had saved the day, and after that Misti went out only when she was well covered and drenched in sun-block.

One night it began to rain as we were sitting on the porch after supper, and as the wind rose, we could feel the raindrops hit us. Misti started to laugh at the feel of the cool rain on her legs. Eager to prolong her pleasure, I moved her to the steps, and together we sat in the rain, experiencing together something most people take for granted—the delicious sensation of water running down our faces, our hair wet and heavy on our shoulders, and our clothes plastered to our bodies. Once, we heard a neighbor scream, "Get that child in out of the rain! Are you crazy?" We just looked at each other and smiled. The crazy people in this world are the ones who do not stop to smell the flowers or feel the raindrops.

Even though she was always busy during the day, we tried to teach Misti that relaxation, too, is a part of life. Sometimes, we sat on the dock and just watched the water in the Chesapeake Bay. Many times Misti was too tired to hold a conversation, but sometimes she would ask about things she did not understand—relationships and people or even physical phenomena. It was almost like revisiting her childhood, especially the weeks and months when "Why?" was a constant question. She asked questions like "Does rain sound the same when it hits water as when it hits the pavement?" When we have all of our senses, we get used to taking in things as a whole and often fail to notice what each sense contributes individually. But when one or another sense is gone or diminished, the others become more acute. At this point, Misti's sight was still so bad that she missed seeing much of what was happening around her, but she used her hearing to compensate. I was constantly amazed at the things she could hear and her interpretation of them.

On those quiet August evenings, we talked about anything and everything—the stars and moon, the tide on the bay, fishing and boating and crabs. On weekends, when Max came over for the evening, we'd all sit out on the porch and talk about the day, about school and friends, and also about Misti's childhood. Even though her long-term memory was better than her short-term memory, Misti seemed to have forgotten a lot, and she needed to hear about Waynesboro in order to remember her life there. Misti drank in every word as I told her and Max about how beautiful she had been as a baby, how smart as a little girl, how she made our family complete, how Chuck and Cork had played with her and the tricks she in turn played on them. Often something I said would lead to a partial memory for her; it was like watching someone sort through a box of old photos, where recognition of one face sparks a memory and further questions.

By the end of the summer, after two and a half months of therapy at Ocean City, Misti's condition had improved immensely. She was using a walker regularly and even taking a few steps on her own, though she still crawled if she was exceptionally tired at the end of the day. Dave Delfanso's work with Misti was clearly helping, and her speech was clear enough for all the therapists and most of the family to understand. Each day continued to have its share of difficulties, but we had begun to see results from everyone's efforts to help Misti learn to control her emotions. Her reasoning was also better, though her attention span was still short.

She was proud of her progress and would occasionally consent to watch the latest videotape. One she day even urged me to videotape her, saying, "Take my picture carrying this to the car!"

As Labor Day approached, Max began to talk about going back to start his senior year of school in Gaithersburg. Since many of the therapists would soon be going back to school as well, we had to make plans to migrate north and set up the same therapies for the continuation of Misti's rehabilitation in Waynesboro.

As at Bryn Mawr, saying good-bye to the people who had become such an important part of our lives in Ocean City was difficult. But while I felt some sadness at having to leave Ocean City, it was overwhelmed by happy anticipation of what the future might hold once we returned to Waynesboro. That was where I grew up, where I went to school, where I was married and worked for twenty-nine years. After more than half a year away from home, I was looking forward to being back on my own turf—Waynesboro, a friendly town where there were few strangers.

Twelve

After the Labor Day weekend, Harry came down to the shore to help with the move. Once again the car would be full. We'd have to haul back the computer, as well as the wheelchair, walker, all the physical therapy equipment, and Misti's clothes and special sneakers. Both Harry's car and mine were loaded, and Max had his packed to the top, too. As we said good-bye to neighbors, Misti started to laugh the all-too-familiar, out-of-control laugh that was the reminder of the accident and brain trauma. Max left and Harry followed, both cars looking like moving vans. Misti and I brought up the rear of the caravan, crammed into a car so full that we couldn't fit in one more stuffed toy, let alone another person. Misti promptly fell asleep, leaving me to negotiate the highway on my own.

When Misti awoke from her nap, she wanted to know where we were going. I told her, and she began asking questions about Waynesboro, about what our home was like, about how she would spend her time. Clearly, she had little recollection of having been back to the house in June or of our numerous discussions over the summer. I reminded her what the house was like and explained that her routine would be similar to those she'd had in Ocean City and Bryn Mawr in many ways.

The four-hour car trip wore on Misti, even before we got to the Bay Bridge. As she became restless, she became angry, and before long, she tried to open the car door and jump out and was kept inside the car only by her seatbelt and shoulder harness. Terror overtook me. I did not like driving over the Bay Bridge under any circumstances, let alone with Misti acting up, but I had no choice. The bridge was within sight, and there was no room for me to pull over to the side of the road. Using my most commanding voice, I told Misti she had to stop her childish behavior immediately. After a summer of hearing profanity, I found my vocabulary affected as well. Now I said, "Shut your damn mouth and keep quiet. I do not like driving over this bridge anyway, and your shit will only make it worse. In fact, if you move a muscle before we get to the other side, you are risking getting the worst beating you can imagine, and I am not joking." I clutched the steering wheel with both sweat-soaked hands, asking God to keep her quiet and calm until we got across the bridge, and Misti fell silent.

When I looked over, after crossing the bridge, it was to find her peacefully asleep, which only took the edge off my shame for having lost my temper. However, I was also proud. Here I was—me, the person who had never driven outside the small town of Waynesboro, except perhaps to Chambersburg or Hagerstown—driving not only across the Bay Bridge, but negotiating the beltway around Washington after a summer of caring for my brain-injured daughter. I felt real pride in my accomplishments and smiled to myself as I remembered Harry's mother saying, "Something good comes out of everything."

Once we arrived at home, our freedom was short-lived. We would need physical, speech, and occupational therapists as well as tutors, doctors, and a facilitator. A phone call from Cathy told me that ACT was still on the case, and only hours passed before therapists started to call. Though she had done a great job in setting up the staff in Ocean City, I once again found myself fearful of the effect of all the changes on Misti.

I thought I knew almost everyone in Waynesboro, but Cathy had clearly gone into high gear in order to find full-time therapists in or near Waynesboro, and she had succeeded in finding some terrific people, including a few I'd never met or even heard of. The only position she had not yet filled was that of speech therapist, and at once Kay Yaukey came to mind. I had known Kay and her husband since the early sixties. Kay was one of the most poised women I had ever known; not only had she sung professionally for years, but her impeccable speech had helped her land many acting jobs both nationally and at the local summer stock theater in Caledonia, just a few miles north of Waynesboro. Most importantly, she knew and liked Misti, and Misti returned the compliment. I thought it would be a great match.

After speaking to Cathy, I walked through the house, taking stock. Time away had certainly taken its toll on my once well-kept home. True, Harry had been using the house, but only the bedroom, bath, and kitchen. He had done a wonderful job of keeping laundry done, and the kitchen and master bedroom and bath were impeccably tidy, but the cleaning lady had quit months ago and not been replaced. I cringed as I noticed dead houseplants with their brown, dried-up leaves. Opening the door to the family room, I watched a moth flicker through the air and shook my head, thinking of the wool oriental rugs. And I got a major surprise when several hundred bees greeted me as I opened the door to the day room. Warm tears fell from my eyes; I had always taken great pride in my home. As I continued to explore, I detected an odor outside the door to the den. When I opened the door, I found the suitcases we'd packed before leaving the Caribbean back in February. Our friends had gathered up our belongings, and into the luggage went wet bathing suits and conch shells (with animals still intact), along with formal evening wear. When I got the suitcases open, I lifted out unrecognizable shreds of rotting clothing and holiday souvenirs. But there was no time for crying over spilled milk. Changing into jeans, I got started on the cleanup, getting groceries, and greeting friends and neighbors. While I was cleaning, Harry was busy making the few simple modifications we would need to get the house set up for Misti: moving furniture to make room for equipment, adding rails to the toilets, and putting a bench in the shower stall.

The local newspaper, *The Record Herald,* wanted to interview Misti and let the town know she was finally home. The reporter had been a schoolmate of Misti's at Mercersburg, and Misti was happy to answer her questions. She insisted on sitting for the picture in the living room, her hair and makeup carefully done, and she made sure that the photo was taken from her good side, so no one would notice that she still had some facial paralysis.

In the photograph taken for the paper, Misti looked normal, and from the interview it seemed that she had made a miraculous recovery from the coma. Someone reading the article on Misti in the newspaper would have no way of knowing about the slurred speech; the walker or the wheelchair; the lost emotions and emotional seizures; or the endless rounds of doctors visits, therapy, and hard work that were Misti's lot to endure if she was to have any kind of normal life. It was not all illusion, of course. Misti *was* making a good and even miraculous recovery. But brain trauma is deceptive. Patients with brain trauma often look quite normal. At Bryn Mawr, they are called "the walking wounded" for that very reason. Because they look so normal, their difficult behavior comes off as even more bizarre. More often than not, they are judged to be nasty, obstinate, or drunk.

◎

In our absence, life in Waynesboro had gone on as usual. As I joined Harry in our old activities and began seeing our friends on a regular basis again, I felt almost as though I had dropped into a time warp. I was surprised how much everything seemed the same, while Misti and I had gone through such tremendous change and upheaval. Perhaps it was my demeanor, perhaps that article in the newspaper, but few people seemed to understand how complicated our lives had become. Friends asked about Misti, but their questions indicated that they thought everything was back to normal at our house.

One Wednesday evening, a facilitator came in to stay with Misti, and Harry and I went out to the Elks Club for dinner with some friends. Across the room, I spied a man who looked familiar and seemed to think I did, too. I clawed through my memory, trying to remember who he was. Then I had it. He smiled as my lips formed his name, "Ben?" The nod of his head catapulted me from my chair, across the room, and into his waiting arms. Ben was just the person I needed now. He had been our family doctor and friend when the boys were young and saw our family through many childhood diseases as well as through my many miscarriages.

As we compared notes on losing hair and gaining weight, his living in France and Hawaii and becoming a grandparent, I mentioned Misti. Knowing that I could not have any more children, he was totally surprised to hear of her existence. I explained about the adoption and then went on to tell him about the accident. He listened patiently and offered to help in any way he could. Once again I marveled at the role fate plays in our lives. Just when we needed him, here was Ben with his great store of knowledge, back in Pennsylvania after being away for over twenty years. When we had a more detailed discussion later, Ben suggested I phone a Dr. Siebens at Good Samaritan Hospital in Baltimore, and he became our new physiatrist, eventually taking over as team leader and director of Misti's rehabilitation.

Visiting Dr. Siebens's office for the first time brought back memories of the rehab up at Paoli. Some of the patients in his waiting room were totally incapacitated. One was lying on a gurney-type table, able to move only his head. Another patient sat in a wheelchair controlled by a tube in his mouth. Some patients were still breathing through tracheostomies. At first glance, Misti seemed physically perfect in comparison to the others in the waiting room. But as we have learned over and over again, one can never imagine what it is like for each patient, behind closed doors.

Cathy had been successful in locating a psychiatrist in Chambersburg, and Misti began making the weekly thirty-minute trip to his office for the hour-long appointment. Dr. Anderson never had a lot to say to me, but since Cathy Cosgrove had found him for us through ACT, I assumed he was knowledgeable about the effects of brain trauma. And Misti seemed to get along with him well enough.

Bryn Mawr Rehab was still involved in Misti's recovery that fall, as the doctors and therapists there evaluated Misti and made recommendations. However, once we met Dr. Siebens, he started running the show. At his direction, Misti and I spent endless days consulting various medical specialists—neurologists, neuro-ophthalmologists, et cetera.—in an effort to discover what the next steps in Misti's recovery should be. The nurse from the CAT fund always accompanied us, tagging along to certify that all of Misti's appointments with these specialists were accident-related. Meanwhile, Harry continued to work hard in order to pay for the doctor bills that the CAT fund refused to cover. We found ourselves heaving deep sighs of relief whenever the fund did pick up a bill or reimburse us for bills that we had paid.

It was through the help of a wonderful man, attorney Robert Michael of Rockville, Maryland, who became our insurance advisor, that we were able to locate many of these specialists and get the CAT fund and our supplemental insurance to pick up the inevitable bills. Many of these specialists occupied rarefied worlds of their own. Because the work these doctors did was so specialized, delicate, and time-consuming, they could pick and choose which patients to take on. Whenever we consulted a new doctor, we had to go through Misti's whole history, and it often felt as if we were auditioning for help.

Almost immediately, Dr. Siebens suggested that we seek out the services of a seizure control specialist for Misti. With help from Robert Michael, we arranged for an appointment for an eight-hour EEG, covering both waking and sleeping hours, at Georgetown University Hospital. Working with the data from that brain study, the seizure control specialists were able to reduce the dosage of Misti's antiseizure medication. Almost immediately, she was more alert, required less sleep, and seemed to learn more quickly.

Every three weeks, Misti, the CAT fund nurse, and I—I was starting to think of us as the Three Musketeers, though it often felt as if we weren't all on the same side—traveled to Good Samaritan Hospital in Baltimore to see Dr. Siebens. He recommended more computer programs to help in Misti's cognitive retraining therapy and wrote countless prescriptions for the therapies and facilitators. The trips were time-consuming, but Misti's recovery continued, so I was not about to argue with the state again about the inefficiency of this process.

When we got to the point of considering Misti's vision, the CAT fund nurse suggested that we consult an eye specialist in northern Pennsylvania. According to this doctor, Misti needed to be fitted with prism glasses and new contact lenses because she was seeing double. As we knew, the situation was complicated because her eyes had been knocked askew in the accident, and she could no longer line images up horizontally. The doctor told us that Misti would need to spend a month at his clinic to learn to use the contact lenses-prism glasses combination. It was now November; if we acted immediately to get her fitted and start the training, she would return home in time for Christmas. Misti was very upset at this news because she would not be able to see Max, who lived too far away to visit often. She would also be away from us for the first time since the accident. Still, she very much wanted to see better, and knowing that time was short, she reluctantly agreed to go.

Just as we were completing the necessary arrangements, a friend suggested that we call the Wilmer Eye Clinic at Johns Hopkins Hospital. A neuro-ophthalmologist there informed us that it should not take Misti an entire month to learn to use prisms. Taking one step back to make those crucial two steps forward, we found ourselves canceling plans for Misti to go to northern Pennsylvania and making a new set of appointments in Baltimore.

After three appointments at the Wilmer Clinic, Misti was fitted with contacts and prism glasses. Shortly thereafter she experienced the thrill of being able to see moderately clearly again. The doctors explained that although the heavy prisms were certainly not the most comfortable way to see, they would improve her vision. Furthermore, the combination of a lowered Tegretol dosage and the new eye equipment should give her better balance and more success walking. Dr. Neil Miller, an eye specialist among eye specialists, would watch Misti's eyes and devise special muscle exercises to help her adjust to the prisms. Then, when he felt the time was right, he would perform surgery, realigning her eyes and doing his best to restore her vision to the way it had been before the accident.

Once we had a rehab team, we held team meetings roughly every month to six weeks. All the therapists attended, as did the reps from ACT, and our new family doctor, Dr. Greg Lyon/Loftus, who kept tabs on Misti's Tegretol levels and watched out for other basic physical problems, such as drug interactions. Dr. Lyon/Loftus was not an expert on brain trauma, but he was a very good doctor, and his attitude was terrific. Since Misti was his patient, he made it his business to learn everything he could about brain trauma so he could be of real help. As our local liaison with Dr. Siebens, he watched for anything important about Misti's condition he thought we should bring to the physiatrist's attention. We'd review what was working, what wasn't, what might help, and which direction to take next.

A normal day for Misti that fall included four to six hours of therapy or doctor's appointments. Misti was getting less rest, but after the Tegretol dosage had been adjusted, she was less tired. Furthermore, the number of emotional storms she experienced in a given week was slowly dropping—probably the result of the continued healing of her brain and her greater distance from Max.

Since he was back at school in Gaithersburg, Max could only see Misti on weekends and maybe one other night a week, because the drive took an hour each way. Like other high school seniors, Max had a busy academic schedule, and after the previous spring's disruptions, his parents wanted him to be home studying more. Thus, the fall was a period of adjustment for Misti and Max. They were separated for longer periods of time, and they were both changing and growing, but in very different directions. Sometimes they got along fine, but there were still a lot of fireworks. They spoke on the phone each evening, and Misti got angry when I tried to limit the calls to no more than half an hour at a time. Often she got upset when Max talked to her about school; she was realizing that Max had a life apart from hers, with other friends, and the only emotion that she could access was anger. She was aware that she had not fully recovered yet, and she was very vulnerable emotionally.

In January, I started taking Misti to Mercersburg so that she could fulfill the required classroom time in English. The long trip was tedious, and I was happy to turn over the chore of driving to the facilitators. Even though we felt that the Academy was being terribly strict about this requirement, we cooperated because we all wanted Misti to get the diploma she'd earned. Once Misti was at the Academy, she didn't have much contact with other students; the rehab team and the staff at Mercersburg had agreed that she wasn't yet ready to attend and participate in a regular class with other students, and so Misti usually sat alone in a classroom, reading what the teachers suggested and putting in the time. Sometimes Mr. Jones, the chaplain, stopped in to chat with Misti, which helped keep her spirits up.

Even when Misti was going to Mercersburg, therapies continued. Some of it was strictly related to the physical recovery from the accident, as when Misti worked with physical therapist Neno Breeno to improve her balance and leg strength, or when she worked on the computer with one her cognitive retraining therapists. But some of the therapy was more involved with life skills, such as helping Misti with her grooming, or putting in her contact lenses, or helping her learn to plan ahead. The occupational therapist, the facilitators, and I worked with Misti on meal planning, shopping, cooking, and in reintroducing her to the community at a speed that she could manage. Not for the first time, I was glad we lived in a small town. For instance, when I took Misti to the bank to open a checking account in her own name, it was a friendly operation. Most of the tellers were young girls who knew Misti, and they were always happy to say hello and spend a few minutes with her. Since we were long-time customers, I was also able to arrange it so that if Misti overdrew her account by a small amount, the bank would transfer money from my account rather than bounce a check and upset her. I can't imagine how we'd have handled this in a bigger city.

I especially appreciated the friendliness of our friends, neighbors, and acquaintances, who always had a smile and a friendly word for Misti. She might otherwise have been lonely since all of her close friends from Waynesboro and Mercersburg were away at college or working during the day. Misti was also getting reintegrated back into family life. She went with me to visit my parents several times a week, and she also went along when we went to see Harry's mother or Uncle Ora and Aunt Goldie. She was getting reacquainted with her nieces and nephews too—especially Victor, the youngest, whose birth six weeks before the accident had somehow been erased from her memory during the coma.

One year and four months after the accident, after finally fulfilling the classroom time that Mercersburg Academy insisted upon, Misti attended a second graduation ceremony and got a real Academy diploma to replace the certificate she'd gotten the previous year. Most of Misti's closest friends had graduated the year before, and she did not seem to recognize many of the other students. As we left the ceremony, we were stopped by Melvin Stewart, a handsome young man with hopes of winning an Olympic gold medal in swimming. When I pushed Misti's wheelchair in his direction, he handed her a booklet with his picture on the front, hugged her, and told her that he would be back to sign it when he won the gold. And in fact, he did win gold in the 1992 Olympic Games.

The entire family was very proud of Misti for having come so far in her rehabilitation. All through the spring, as it was apparent that her recovery was progressing. Harry, Misti, and I had been talking about where she might go to further her education. Misti was excited about going on to college, as all her friends had done, and though we spent a lot of time talking about the many new challenges this would represent, we saw no reason to discourage her.

The colleges she had been accepted by two years before were not holding places for her, and she was likely to have a very hard time fitting in and keeping up at a regular four-year college. We explained all this to Misti and pointed out that it would be easier and more practical if she went to a community college or to the Penn State school in nearby Mont Alto. We also talked about the fact that at first she would be going to classes with a facilitator and be in a wheelchair, becoming more independent as time went on. We always reached for the stars as far as Misti's recovery was concerned, knowing that we were stretching our hopes and even dreaming dreams. But by this time, Misti was becoming more confident and looking forward to continued challenges and further progress. And though she was becoming aware of her deficits through ever greater exposure to a wider world, this was not as harmful as it would have been earlier. As Misti was getting ready to take on more of life, Harry and I did our best to guide her; beyond that, we could only pray and hope for the best.

The summer of 1989 was very busy with therapies aimed at getting Misti ready for college. She did a lot of work with her physical therapist, Neno Breeno, who was just a super person. Although he was very busy and his office was about forty-five minutes away, we didn't have to make the trip; instead, he came to our home for Misti's therapy. I sometimes cringed as I watched him make Misti balance on a sheet of plywood that teetered like a see-saw. Still, the results were impressive. The prism glasses and the drop in her dose of Tegretol had really made a difference and helped improve her balance markedly. By the time she was ready to go to Mont Alto that fall, she was able to take some steps unassisted, even though she would continue to use the wheelchair to get between classes. But in time, she was able to leave the chair behind, stop using her walker, and later abandon her cane.

Misti also continued working with Kay Yaukey. Kay was the first person who had ever really been able to overcome Misti's objections and get her to try to sing. She was confident that singing would give more inflection to Misti's rather monotone voice, which sounded almost like a robot's or the telephone company's automated information service. Though her speech was sometimes unrecognizable to people who didn't know her, especially when she was tired, it was understandable to the people working with her, and with Kay's work each week, it showed steady improvement.

The computer, too, was a great aid, helping not only to improve Misti's cognitive functions as she did formal exercises and learned the strategy of games, but also her fine-motor-skills as she typed on the keyboard. Over the summer, we needed to have fewer team meetings, and the frequency of the various therapies dwindled from every day to only three or four times a week for each.

Of course, Max had graduated from high school in June as well, and though Misti did not attend the graduation ceremony, we did take her down to the Greys' house for the party afterward. However, that summer marked the beginning of the end of their relationship. Max and Misti continued to spend time together, but it was increasingly clear that Max was getting ready to move on. Tension between them seemed to be growing. Misti was very jealous of any time Max spent away from her, and when he left Waynesboro to go home to Gaithersburg, she often got unruly. No amount of reasoning could persuade her that her possessiveness was pushing him away. Instead, she told me that the problem was that I did not understand modern relationships, that I was still living in the fifties.

When Misti started at Mont Alto in September, she was a day student taking only a few classes, and all her therapies continued, though with less intensity than before. She was able to walk on her own within the buildings, but she used a wheelchair on campus, and either I or a facilitator accompanied her everywhere. Fortunately, Mont Alto, like Waynesboro, was something of an extended family for us. Harry had done a lot of construction work on campus, and I had decorated the offices and homes of some of the college's faculty and administration, so they knew us well and were sympathetic to Misti's situation. By and large, people at Mont Alto were very welcoming to Misti, and I knew that friends on campus could be counted on to keep a watchful eye out for her and provide a safety net if need be.

Misti found the early days of college exciting, exhausting, and sometimes confusing. On the days a facilitator took her to campus, I always got a lot of phone calls from her, and I tried to be reassuring. But even with all of our careful preparations, it was a lot for Misti to take on at once. The situation with Max added another layer of complications to the volatile mix.

Max was attending college near Virginia Beach, some five hours away from Waynesboro, and the commute was not easy. Though Misti seemed steadier emotionally in the summer, having fewer outbursts a week, she was still taking Tegretol to safeguard against seizures, and any contact with Max seemed to provoke upset. Once he went away to school, Misti seemed to regress emotionally, having more and more intense emotional storms as September went on. Perhaps because I was the person closest to Misti on an everyday basis, I was the target of many of them.

As her emotional behavior became more and more erratic, I became worried. So, I was especially happy when near the end of September, Dr. Anderson, who almost never called, phoned to say that he would like to see me, alone. He told me that he had just discovered the source of Misti's outbursts and uncontrollable behavior, and he wanted to share his breakthrough with me. Terrific, I thought; now we could really move forward.

As I went into Dr. Anderson's office, I was sure that I was about to learn what was causing Misti's emotional regression and how we could deal with it. Settling myself across from his scarred desk, I leaned forward to hear his explanation, prepared to absorb his every word. Then I got a big surprise. "The reason for Misti's outbursts," he stated, "is anger." I continue to listen. "Anger at you"—this sounded reasonable enough to me—"and her father because she is adopted."

At that, I sprang to my feet, furious. "Because she is *adopted*? Excuse me, doctor, but don't you realize that this girl was hit by a tractor trailer, her head split open, her brain exploded from its skull, and that she's been through months of rehabilitative therapy? And now you're telling me that she is upset because she is adopted?" I turned, stalked out, and managed to get into my car before I screamed, "You crazy nut! You insensitive, insane bastard! All this time wasted."

Driving home, I realized I had to call Cathy Cosgrove at ACT. We had to find a new psychiatrist—a competent doctor this time. When I got home, I found Misti and her current facilitator in an argument that resembled fireworks on the Fourth of July. Thirty minutes later, realizing I was now without either a facilitator or a psychiatrist, I sat down to try to talk to Misti. After I got her calmed down, I explained to her that we would have to find new people to fill the voids. She vehemently refused to see another psychiatrist, explaining to me that they all were crazy. She advised me to take a look at the many we had consulted since the accident, "none of which had helped anyway." It was a telling moment. How could I argue with her reasoning? Even with brain trauma she had enough intelligence to realize that we had only been spinning our wheels.

Still, we couldn't give up. From all I knew about rehabilitation after brain trauma, it was clear that a good psychiatrist—a knowledgeable, compassionate professional who could help patients make sense of the changes in their lives and who could point out problems while offering encouragement that recovery was possible—was essential. And if it was up to me to locate such a person, so be it. As my fingers did the walking through the Yellow Pages, they came across a familiar name: Dr. Harvey Shapiro. Misti and I knew Dr. Shapiro from Mercersburg Academy, where he had been the psychiatrist available to the academic community. The Academy made a big point of making sure students were comfortable with all of the staff so they would not hesitate to get help should they need it, and Dr. Shapiro was familiar with all of the students. Though he was a general psychiatrist with no special expertise in brain trauma, I was able to persuade a reluctant Misti to let me call him. He had known her before, I responded. He might be in a better position to help now.

When I called Cathy Cosgrove to set it up, however, she explained that payment for his services would be up to us because Dr. Shapiro was not one of the doctors on the CAT fund list. I interrupted, "You mean to tell me we can only go to doctors chosen by CAT? Because of the way the system is set up, if I take my daughter to a knowledgeable doctor who might actually be able to help, we have to pay for it out of our own pockets?" She agreed that this was the case.

I began to realize just how the system worked. After all the red tape was neatly wound on its spools, the situation was this: Under the auspices of the CAT fund, all drivers paid mandatory fees and were covered by the state insurance pool—but only to see a CAT-authorized doctor. It was like being forced to join a restrictive HMO. If you drove, you had to pay the fees, but you could go to only certain doctors, and if the doctor who might be able to help was not on the list, you were out of luck, or at least, out of pocket. And maddeningly, while they might not pay for a local doctor who could help Misti, they did continue to pay for a CAT fund nurse to leave Harrisburg, drive to Waynesboro, follow us in her car to every long-distance specialist's appointment. She would sit in the waiting room with us, listen to the entire appointment with pen and clip board in hand and ask at the end, "Was everything the Morningstars talked to you about accident-related?" When the doctor answered the obvious "Yes," she checked the proper square on her clipboard and followed us on the drive back to make sure we didn't stop anywhere else. The state would pay a nurse's salary and mileage for two cars, but not for a visit to Dr. Shapiro because he wasn't on their list.

When I once suggested to the nurse that it might be more efficient to wait at her desk in Harrisburg and ask the doctor to call her at the end of our visit to answer the same question, she merely said, "That's not the way we do it." It probably made sense from her perspective: When she accompanied us down to Baltimore for appointments and tests, she got paid for ten to eleven hours a day. But, in that amount of time, it seemed to me, she could sit in her office for eight hours, talk on the phone to ten doctors, and make ten check marks. At the very least, her mileage would be cut to less than half. Taking into account the number of patients she worked with, this savings would allow the fund to use doctors outside of the CAT network.

Even an uneducated person like myself could understand why the CAT fund had been abolished a few months before. (We had been assured that the fund would continue to take care of patients injured before and covered under the fund.) Harry and I decided that the CAT fund payment policy would not change things for Misti. I would continue to search out the best care for her, and Harry would continue to work to be able to pay for what she needed.

What Misti needed help with just now was in coping with the changing situation with Max. As soon as the semester had started, Misti realized that he would be visiting Waynesboro even less often than before, and she got more and more upset about this. She began to realize that Max's world had widened considerably, and she was not as big a part of it. He was having a different experience than she was: Going to college out of state and living in a dorm was just not the same as going to school six miles away from home while living with your parents. Now when Max called, he was telling Misti about his wider world. She heard about all his new adventures, from the classes to the parties, from the free-and-easy dorm situation to the many new female friends he was making . The name Mary Anna started to come up in his conversation very frequently. Misti did not pick up on Max's interest in Mary Anna immediately, but before too long, the two of them were having phone arguments that left her screaming, "You are f—-ing Mary Anna!"

It was not surprising that as a teenager away at school for the first time, Max's horizons had expanded. Nor was it surprising that Misti was very hurt and angry at this turn of events. She was so upset, in fact, that she began to threaten to commit suicide. Though she had always been dramatic in her presentation of problems—after all, this was the same girl who had once threatened to flush her head down the commode if I didn't come and pick her up at Mercersburg immediately—we had to take her threats seriously. Misti used the bathroom alone and had a razor so she could shave her own legs. Her threats could be carried out in only a few minutes. I checked on her frequently, and I asked the facilitator to do the same, but I had to walk a fine line. However worried I was, I did not want to deprive her of her hard-won independence by going back to helping her shower or use the bathroom.

When I called Dr. Shapiro to let him know about Misti's threats and the fact that she had begun lashing out violently at me in ways she hadn't since the summer we'd spent in Ocean City, he agreed that she should come in at once. He had followed Misti's story since the accident and knew that she was recovering from head injury. When Harry and I brought her to Dr. Shapiro's office, he agreed that Misti's emotional state was indeed precarious and suggested a change in the kind of attention and emotional support she was getting. He also felt strongly that it would not be good for either of us if she continued to vent all of her rage over Max's defection at me. He recommended that Misti be admitted to the psychiatric unit of the Chambersburg Hospital for observation, and when we agreed, he took her directly from his office to the nearby hospital, sending Harry and me home to pack a suitcase with Misti's clothes and toiletries. When I returned to the hospital later I watched the attendants check Misti's bag to make sure that all her grooming aids were in clear plastic bottles and that there were no sharp objects. I felt sad, helpless, and almost defeated when they asked me to leave. It was almost as though she were being put in prison.

Misti's breakdown and hospitalization were very hard on us, especially Harry, who always coped best when there was something physical he could do to help. Since the time a Bryn Mawr nurse told Max that he could have inadvertently hurt Misti when he took the initiative to try to help her stand, Harry had always wary of helping with her care without explicit instructions from a professional. He found it frustrating when he could only stand by, watching and waiting but unable to help. It made him restless. As it happened, he was scheduled to leave for a long-planned, long-since-paid-for hunting trip to the wilds of northwestern Canada early the day after Misti was admitted to Chambersburg Hospital. With Misti in the hospital, he felt he couldn't go. After a long discussion, however, we decided that there was nothing to be gained by his staying home; we had been told that Misti might stay in the hospital for several weeks. It was impossible to rearrange the timing of the trip or to get a refund, and it would be a shame to lose the money he had already paid.

After he left the next morning, the house was very quiet. With Harry away, Chuck and Teresa brought Valera and Victor by, and Cork and Jill stopped in with Emily and Betsy to keep me company. But with no Misti, and thus no therapies or facilitators coming or going, the silence was heavy and oppressive. For five days I made the trip to Chambersburg Hospital for visiting hour. Then Misti had a severe emotional outburst, cursing, striking out at me, and screaming that she never wanted to see me again. Dr. Shapiro recommended that I wait for a while before coming back to visit since Misti was continuing to use me as her whipping boy, which would help neither of us. He promised to call when she had calmed down sufficiently for a visit to be productive.

Back home, Max's mother called to check on Misti's condition and was very disturbed to hear of her regression. We also discussed Max for a few minutes. As I hung up, I had the feeling that Max had already made his last visit to our house. I realized that Brenda's tactful words—"Settled in school, Max is so busy with his studies and his new friends that he barely has time for his own family"—really meant was that he would have no more time for Misti. As I stared at the telephone receiver in its cradle, I felt pangs of regret. I fervently wished I had made a stronger stand when Max wanted to live in Ocean City the previous summer. If only I had put my foot down then, Misti would have had to accept an inevitable situation at a point when she was less likely and less able to hurt herself. It would have been difficult, but surely it would have been easier to break the ties to Max then. But it was too late now, and I tried to remind myself of what I have tried to teach Misti: We cannot cry over what might have been.

The days seemed endless as I waited for Misti's state to improve enough to make our visits helpful. In a few days, Dr. Shapiro called to let me know that he was working with Misti and she was calming down, but it was his feeling that Misti would fare better if we stayed apart for a while longer; in the meantime, she would be safe and I would have a rest from her attacks. This was certainly true, but it was a very difficult time for me nonetheless. Harry was away, our new minister was not someone I knew well, and the rest of the family was either preoccupied with their own worries or not sure how to help.

While Misti was in the hospital, I threw my nervous energy into cleaning the house within an inch of its life and spending time with my parents. As my father's life dwindled with the Alzheimer's, he had become an empty shell of a human, drawn into the fetal position and offering no response to any stimulation. He had once built a business, raised a family, been a successful plumbing and heating engineer, and soon he would have to be put into a nursing home where his frail body could be better cared for. It was terribly sad.

Meanwhile, some of the staff at the hospital seemed to be handling Misti's breakdown as if she were the victim of some antifeminist plot. Drawing only on input from Misti, the head nurse wrote the following report: "Because of her bad temper in the past, relatives and family refuse to help take care of her. Mother and patient are enmeshed. Mother has built her own life around this patient. Parents' marriage is very dysfunctional. Mother is trying to avoid being alone and dealing with her own issues. Suspect much of patient's anger outburst are her reaction to this enmeshment."

Over the next several weeks, the reports at the hospital, particularly from the psychiatric ward's militantly feminist head nurse and the social worker, continued to be negative about the way I had handled the situation. Misti's point of view, embraced by these two mental health professionals, who had neither knowledge of the family situation nor expertise in head injury, was that I was the problem because I would not allow her the independence to do what she wanted. Misti told them that my expectations for her were not necessarily her expectations and hopes for herself. This was enough for the nurse and social worker, who were oblivious to the effects of head injury and felt that Misti should move into her own apartment, start driving again, and get on with her life in the manner of her own choice. Furthermore, they said, if it was Misti's desire to conduct multiple short-term sexual relationships with male friends, then that was her choice, and it should not be the business of her family.

At this point, Dr. Shapiro cut this absurdly ideological discussion short and brought everyone back to reality. When he discussed with Misti the idea of getting her own apartment, she herself admitted that she didn't think the plan would work out. She had calmed down considerably and realized that she might not be able to do everything necessary to live on her own. When Dr. Shapiro asked her if she would place an ad in the newspaper to find a facilitator to help with the living arrangements, Misti couldn't manage even this step. With that, the staff at the hospital decided that perhaps Misti could not handle so much independence.

Once again, we found ourselves in the position of having to deal with people who were not educated about brain damage. And again, the people in question were mental health professionals who had leapt into a situation without fully understanding it. Many people, including the ward's head nurse and social worker, did not seem to realize that there are significant differences between the mental and emotional problems caused by brain trauma and those caused by a chemical imbalance or even neurosis. No matter what they believed about dysfunction in the Morningstar family or the place of the emancipated female in the world, the fact was that Misti had suffered brain trauma, and the results of brain trauma are not easily corrected.

Everything seemed so simple to them, all situations either deepest black or purest white, with no intervening shades of gray. Perhaps because of years of working as an interior designer, my eye was trained to see many shades of gray. Maybe Misti and I had grown too close, but that was the result of the accident and its aftermath, not something else. After all, until the accident, Misti had lived away from home and was planning to go away to college with my blessing. When she was well enough to go away to school or live on her own, I would be more than happy to let her go. It was true that other young women her age were making independent decisions about their sexual activity, but those young women had not been through a terrible accident, deep coma, or extensive rehabilitation. When it came to the nurse's and social worker's therapeutic insight into Misti's problems, I had the all too familiar sinking feeling that we were going nowhere fast. However, they did keep her safe, and that was important.

Perhaps they we were right about one aspect of the situation: If Misti and I were able to spend more time apart, she would be better able to cope with her situation. For Misti, a big part of that would be getting her driver's license back. Even though I was concerned about her continued emotional outbursts and what might happen if she had such an outburst while driving, I promised that we would work toward that goal. In the meantime, Misti would spend more time with facilitators and less time with me. I would try to give her more space, allow her to do her own laundry and cook meals. She could work toward independence and perhaps in the near future move into an apartment on her own.

Once the issue of Misti's growth toward independence was settled, the hospital staff turned to the problem of her breakup with Max. She could learn to deal with this, they felt, by reading a book on the subject. Of course, Dr. Shapiro and I both knew that it would be more complicated than that, requiring ongoing therapy and a slow, steady rebuilding of her self-confidence.

After several weeks in the hospital, Misti was ready to be discharged and return home with me. As I got ready to pick her up at the hospital, I collected the postcards Harry had sent from his hunting trip and drove the familiar highway to the hospital, finally stepping through the doors to the psychiatric unit. When Misti saw me, she reached out her arms for a tight hug. Before we left, she introduced me to the new friends she had made while at the hospital.

It was great to have her back home. Harry was delighted to hear about Misti's release. He called several times to check on her progress and to give us updates on his hunt. Misti went back to classes at Mont Alto and started spending more time with facilitators as we had planned. Life went on, pretty much normally. However, the month she'd spent in hospital had put her behind in her classes, and Misti had to drop first one class, then another.

Once she was over the worst of the upset at her breakup with Max, Misti began to make progress again. But the brain takes its own time to heal, and troubles kept brewing. We had all been warned by Dr. Shapiro to be careful about the television programs Misti watched, because she was still having difficulty distinguishing truth from fantasy and sometimes confused real life with the sensational stuff she saw on TV. Dr. Shapiro had been careful to stress that Misti should absolutely not be allowed to watch soap operas, no matter how much she begged. With all the confusion in her mind about relationships, she certainly did not need to be exposed to stories about women having affairs with other people's husbands or parents molesting their children and so on. We always screened the movies she watched before letting her see them, yet even the plots of movies we'd screened sometimes caused problems.

One morning not long after she'd been released from the hospital, Misti accused me of sleeping with Max as recently as two weeks before, while she had been in the hospital. She also accused me of having slept with him at the hotel in Paoli when she was at Bryn Mawr and questioned me about her having been sexually abused when she was a small child. Of course, none of this had happened; there had never been a time that this could have happened, and I explained that to her. She insisted that I did not know as much as I thought I did. I was always firm with her in my replies, but her questions went around and around in my mind to the point that I almost began to doubt my own sanity.

Then one afternoon, when I arrived home earlier than expected, I heard the TV playing and realized that Misti and the current facilitator had been watching *General Hospital*. I was furious, of course, and I made it clear to the facilitator. But my anger did not help the situation, and soon I found we needed to hire a new facilitator. Again, Cathy Cosgrove would have to find someone to fill the void. Finding a good facilitator was not always easy. Though the job wasn't skilled per se—the most important qualification was getting along with Misti—the person had to have some initiative and lots of common sense. Sometimes we were lucky and sometimes we were not. This had been one of our unlucky phases.

For the next few days, I had a friend tape *General Hospital* for me to watch after Misti was in bed. Never having watched the soaps, I found the world of daytime dramas a revelation. I got a real education, and I had to wonder how exposure to this stuff was affecting small children who were at home during the day. In just a little time, I knew how it had been affecting Misti: The accusations she had been making were taken straight out of the plot of the TV show. We redoubled our efforts to keep track of what she was watching. In an effort to avoid some of these confusions, Dr. Shapiro suggested that instead of having a facilitator drive her to their weekly sessions, I start bringing Misti to his office so that he could talk first with Misti and then with both of us together. This strategy was sometimes successful, allowing Misti to make progress and me to figure out better ways of coping, but sometimes, like many things connected with brain injury, it was no help at all.

❧

By November, Dr. Miller at the Wilmer Clinic had changed Misti's monthly appointments to biweekly visits in anticipation of the operation on her eyes. The great day arrived a few days before Christmas. Our grandson Victor's birthday celebration was put on hold as Harry and I took Misti down to Johns Hopkins. Dr. Miller performed the surgery early in the morning, and the operation to realign her eyes went well. Interestingly, Dr. Miller corrected the problem with Misti's vision by realigning the muscles of the "good" right eye to correspond with the "bad" left eye, rather than vice versa. Misti left the operating room in good condition, with Dr. Miller planning to adjust the sutures six hours after the surgery.

True to his word, Dr. Miller returned later that day to take Misti to another room, and Harry and me were allowed to go along. Misti sat in a chair resembling an old-fashioned dentist chair, and he removed the gauze bandages from her eyes and revealed a long black thread hanging over her cheek. With a light in front of her, he pulled on the string to tighten the muscles and then gave it slack until she cried out, "I can see, I can see." The smile on her face was quickly replaced by a look of disappointment, though. Dr. Miller explained that the surgery had caused swelling and she would not be able to see well for a short while longer. He assured us that he had done a magnificent job and that she would be fine. However, because of the damage done in the accident, she would always have to wear glasses, which would not be thin or lightweight. He gave me a list of instructions on how to care for her until we returned for her next office visit. On the bottom of the paper, he had written out his phone numbers by hand—his private numbers at the office and at home—and he told us we could call at any time.

As the family prepared for Christmas in 1989, Misti was frustrated because she could not see with any consistency. She could not be part of the all the pre-Christmas activities, like baking or wrapping presents, and Harry and I were at our wits' end to keep her comfortably occupied. Because her eye was healing from the operation, the usual time-passers and distractions did not work: She could not focus well enough to play games on the computer, and though she could read for very brief periods of time with an eye patch, or watch MTV, ultimately the eye fatigue would overcome her. She would listen to the radio or her Walkman for awhile but then get bored. Harry and I both tried to keep her amused, but much of the time, she was understandably miserable. Each day I prayed that the next would be better.

But her vision problems didn't keep Misti from recovering in other ways. One day was particularly memorable. Donna Kaufman, the wonderful new facilitator ACT had found after the fiasco with the soap opera fan, had left for the day, and I was doing the last thing on the day's lengthy to-do list: trying out a new recipe for a Lady Baltimore cake that my sister-in-law Beck had given me. As I tried to frost the cake, the layers slid first to one side then to the other, and Misti laughed as I moaned and complained. Finally, in desperation, I took the cake outside into the cold and put it on a table on the patio to try to harden the icing and keep the cake in place.

While I was outside, a bored and mischievous Misti succeeded in dialing Beck's phone number. "Aunt Beck, Mom is in trouble." "What happened?" "The cops came and took her away." "Oh my God, what happened?" "I'm not sure," Misti continued, "something about murder." "Oh my God! No! Misti, listen to me. Are *you* all right?" "Yes." "Is anyone with you?" "No." "Where is your dad?" "I don't know." "Is he okay?" "I think so." "Now listen to me, sit down and stay where you are. Uncle Dave and I will be there in a few minutes".

Then with a devilish tone, Misti's voice cooed into Beck's ear, "Oh, don't bother, she only killed Lady Baltimore." Then she giggled and hung up the phone.

The phone was ringing as I walked in the door, and I picked it up to find a nearly hysterical Beck on the line. Everything was quite fine, except for the cake, I explained, and Beck stammered out that this had been the most traumatic thing that ever happened to her since she had started nurses' training. Knowing all the pressure I had been under, she explained, what with the holidays and all, she was afraid that I had finally cracked. Misti was only exercising her returning sense of humor with a childish prank, but she had touched on a subject that Dave and Beck had talked about fearfully in the privacy of their own home.

☺

Dr. Miller had prescribed medications to help Misti's eye heal faster and prevent infection. However, her eye stayed red, and two days after Christmas, as I prepared to put the ointment in her eye, I noticed a red pimply-looking spot on the eyeball. Fear ripped through me; the eyes are so delicate. The last thing Misti needed to contend with after the turmoil this fall was a new problem with her eye. Quickly, I looked up the numbers Dr. Miller had given me and tried his private office line. Though it was only 7:00 A.M., I got Dr. Miller himself. After I explained the situation, he calmed me down, assuring me that everything would be fine; the pimple was just a reaction from the surgery and would go away if we just kept using the ointment as prescribed.

Still irritable because she could not see, Misti retreated to her room, keeping to herself as much as we permitted. In the early afternoon, I heard her scream, "Mom, quick, Mom." Running with all the speed my fifty-year-old legs could muster, I arrived at her door to hear wonderful news: "Mom, I can see, I can really see. It's wonderful!" A short fifteen minutes later, the sight had faded again, and Misti fell back into gloom.

The same things happened the next day, with Misti's sight lasting for about half an hour; it happened later in the evening as well. These episodes continued for three more days, with each interlude of good vision lasting longer until, finally, Misti's sight returned for good. She was ecstatic, and so were the rest of us. In January we took one more trip back to Wilmer and had contacts fitted, and Misti finally experienced consistently good vision. Fortunately, Misti's occupational therapy had done its job, and Misti could put in the lenses herself. We had to stop and thank God for the wonderful miracles of modern medicine and the doctors who work so diligently to make them happen.

Thirteen

With the new year came a new life for Misti, who would be attending Mont Alto full time. Since we lived only six miles away from the campus and there was a shortage of residential space for noncommuting students, the school was unwilling to give her a dorm room, which made Misti angry. She felt she was now ready to go away to college, and if she couldn't get into a dorm, she wanted to get an apartment and live on her own.

Given her age—she was now nineteen—this seemed quite reasonable. To look at Misti at this point was to behold at a miracle. She looked both attractive and healthy, her face beautiful, her hair glossy and smooth. One only noticed her few remaining deficits when she started to move or speak: She was still unsteady and slow in her movements, with her left hand and leg rather weak, and she occasionally needed to touch a wall or rail for support while walking. Her voice was rather soft and a bit halting, though her speech itself was clear and understandable.

Misti also had a tendency to repeat herself in conversation—a residue of her problems with short-term memory. But she was convinced that she had recovered fully and had no further problems, and she got angry when anyone told her she needed more rehabilitation. She insisted that she needed only physical therapy to work on her walking, which she asserted was the only significant remaining deficit. However, in the judgment of both Drs. Siebens and Lyon/Loftus, she could not yet be left alone because of possible seizure activity—a judgment that was reinforced when Misti told us that she still had episodes of dizziness and fainting-type sensations. She also admitted to having spells when she could not understand what people around her were saying, even when she could see their mouths moving and hear the sounds they made.

Dr. Shapiro spent long hours with her, gently trying to point out the deficits that remained so she would accept them but not become too discouraged to continue to work on them. Throughout that winter and early spring, he reasoned with her about the inadvisability of living alone, pointing out that contact with other people was a very good thing.

My worries about Misti at this time were very concrete. She was still behaving quite seductively and offering open invitations to the young men around her. I was very much afraid that if she were unsupervised, she would be quite vulnerable to men who wouldn't understand her problems and might take advantage of her. Left to live independently, she could be hurt emotionally by some fellow just out for a good time or even become pregnant and be abandoned.

Misti, meanwhile, was feeling somewhat stifled. She didn't want to be closely supervised, she didn't want to live at home any longer, and she didn't want interference from other people, however well-meaning.

Most of all, she insisted that the Commonwealth of Pennsylvania should restore her driver's license. We had had to surrender her license while Misti was still in the STU at Bethesda because that was the legal requirement for all patients with head trauma. Obviously, this had not been an issue while Misti was at Bryn Mawr, in Ocean City, or while she was still finishing up her requirements at Mercersburg. But once she was ready to start college, she wanted to be more independent, and to her that meant having her license.

When Dr. Shapiro explained to her what had happened, she became really angry at the fact that Mr. Winslow, who had caused the accident and the damage to her brain, had been able to keep his license while she had had to give hers up. In the interests of justice, she felt that he should have to surrender his license as well, and there was no way to argue with her on this point. It took her quite some time to get over this, especially since both Dr. Shapiro and I felt that her emotions were still too volatile to make it safe for her to start driving again.

One of her other complaints was that she had to wear supportive sneakers all the time, instead of more fashionable shoes like everyone else on campus. On this, we were happy to try accommodating her. However, when she changed from the sneakers to other shoes, she began to have difficulty walking. When we consulted an orthopedist at Johns Hopkins about this, he explained that Misti had a soft tissue injury of the left foot with some residual scarring. However, he was sure that if she continued to walk as much as possible and kept exercising, she would be able to overcome the problem.

Once we got Misti settled for the new semester, Harry and I were ready for a rest. Unfortunately, within a few days we were once again in the midst of uproar. Because of changes in our family life (we no longer needed so big a house) and the requirements of Harry's new real estate development business, we had put our home up for sale. Since the real estate market was generally rather slow, we had been sure it would be spring before anything happened. As it happened, we were wrong, and the house sold within days. The closing would be quick, so we would have to pack and move quickly, within a matter of weeks. An unsold townhouse in the Morningstar Heights development, which was ready for immediate occupancy, would be our new home.

Moving from a house with all the possessions we had collected in the past thirty-three years would not be easy; we'd have to decide what we'd need in the townhouse and what should go into storage, and then pack everything up. The day after we accepted the buyer's offer, Harry and I started packing. Since we had lived in the house for so long, each room held memories of joys and sorrows, happiness and setbacks. When I surveyed the den and noticed a scar on the solid knotty-white pine wall that Harry had so lovingly finished, I remembered Chuck and Cork's fierce fight over the toy space gun years before. A look around the sun room reminded me of happy hours spent tending plants and companionable hours spent with Misti.

In the new townhouse we'd be giving up significant space and comfort. We'd be going from a house with a dayroom, family room, den, and living room, to a townhouse with only a living room. And having been away from home for so long, it felt as though I had just gotten back. Again, I had to remind myself that what was, was, and what was not, was not. Interestingly, since her memories of the house were no longer so acute, Misti was excited rather than upset at the prospect of moving. Even though her new bedroom would be smaller, she'd be getting a small study and her own bath.

Because Misti did not have classes the next day, she would help supervise the movers' actions around her room. She, too, had had to make decisions about what would be stored. She was particularly concerned that her computer be loaded correctly and not mistreated.

The movers were three young men who definitely had many more muscles than brains. Misti immediately started flirting with one who had long, lank hair, numerous tattoos, and a toothless smile. He was pleasant enough and very friendly, returning the attention she was giving him, but having seen Misti throw herself at young men, I worried. I made sure I kept an eye out during the many trips to Misti's room, and as she moved from flirtation to attempted seduction, the words of the song Elvis made popular ran through my mind: "Lord, you gave me a mountain, this time a mountain too high to climb."

Misti's behavior with the moving men confirmed my opinion that regardless of what the mental health professionals at the hospital in Chambersburg had said, she was not yet ready to be on her own. Because her shaky self-esteem had taken such a blow from Max's painful defection, even living in a dorm could be dangerous. I knew that she was growing up and gaining independence and that we had to let her do so, but I was also conscious of the potential dangers.

After the move, I called Dr. Shapiro to share my concerns. He reminded me that Misti's current problems, ironically, were connected to the fact that she had started out with so much going for her. He said, "Before the accident, Misti was one of the most brilliant young people I have ever met. Her IQ was in the range of 160. She had plans, dreams, and expectations consistent with that. Before the accident she was a ballerina of some accomplishment, and now she cannot walk normally. Not many of us would be able to tolerate losing so much and still be able to function. It's because she was so utterly superior before the accident that she is now able to realize her deficits. There is no way to escape the fact that her life has been profoundly altered. Her problems arise because she very much wants to be accepted by her peers, but due to the accident, she has lost her ability to judge her actions with thought for their consequences."

"Great, Dr. Shapiro," I said. "We know *why* Misti has problems, but what do we do? We can talk about it all day and rationalize about it, but the truth is, if she is not protected from herself, her life could be altered even more."

He was in complete agreement with Harry and me and suggested that Misti's move to a dorm or apartment be postponed until we could see some changes in her behavior. He had to admit that this was a very tough situation, one that we would have to feel our way through carefully. Meanwhile, we would all continue to talk with her about the way young men were likely to respond to her current brand of friendliness.

At the suggestion of Misti's physical therapist, and with the approval of Dr. Shapiro, the fitness club at the edge of town started to occupy many of Misti's free hours. She was now spending forty-eight hours a week with her facilitator Donna, who was a terrific companion for Misti not only because she herself had had to recover from an accident years ago, but also because she looked even closer to Misti's age than her young thirty years. Misti liked Donna a good deal, and Donna, in turn, was devoted to Misti. Each day that spring, she drove her to school, brought her home afterward for a snack, and then took her to the health club, which was run by a friend of Cork's. There, Michael Shockley, the club's trainer, assisted her with the exercises that Neno Breeno had designed to help her with her gait. At the gym, Misti had an opportunity to socialize with other young people in a relatively controlled setting.

As time went on, Misti's life assumed more and more the shape of a healthy young woman's. Since she continued to be so dependent on me, even though she wasn't happy about it, I was happy that she was still spending time with Kay Yaukey. Although she needed less speech therapy, she continued to see Kay on a limited basis, going with her to plays and to the ballet. She admired Kay, and their pleasant excursions meant that she was going out into the world with someone besides members of her family.

Misti had also stayed in close touch with Barbara Patrick, a young woman she had met in the hospital. Barbara and her husband ran a printing business in a neighboring town, and they offered Misti a job for the summer. When I learned about this, I was very happy to know that Misti would be working. Maybe she would begin to feel that she was no longer primarily a patient but instead a capable person who could live a normal life. In addition, she would be making some money and would no longer be dependent on Harry and me for every cent.

Misti's growing independence brought the two of us closer and was accompanied by a decrease in the number and severity of her outbursts and accusations. She still insisted that most of what I said was wrong—especially about dating, since I was "too ancient" to have any real idea how young men and women got along these days—and she was quick to point out my mistakes. However, by the summer of 1990, it had been months since she struck me and a longer time since she had bitten or kicked me. She still needed to have someone keep an eye on her because of her inappropriate displays of sexuality, but I felt sure that as she gained independence and self-respect in other aspects of her life, this would change also. I only prayed to God that nobody took advantage of her vulnerability before her recovery was complete.

As Misti and I drove down to Good Samaritan Hospital to see Dr. Siebens in June 1990, we had our first real mother and daughter chat since the accident. Listening to Misti and seeing her looking so healthy and so calmly self-confident made me realize just how large the strides were that she had taken in the last few months.

Dr. Siebens was pleased with Misti's progress and suggested that she should have a speech/language pathology evaluation, and since Misti was so insistent, a driving evaluation as well. He also suggested that her cognitive retraining be tapered and that physical therapy, occupational therapy, and psychological treatment be changed from twice to once a week. Since Misti was doing so well with spending so much time with Donna, he said we should continue this schedule for the present. In addition, he ordered a neuropsychological assessment be done over the summer. Dr. Siebens gave an okay to Misti's taking a short vacation in the Caribbean accompanied by Donna, which we hoped would give Misti some more experience at functioning apart from me. The recovery of Misti's driver's license would be next on the agenda. He would see her again in one month to see how the tapered rehabilitation program was working out, review the results of the assessment in speech and language, and conduct the driving evaluation.

Misti and I left Dr. Siebens's office glowing with the feelings of accomplishment and success. These days, Misti walked most of the time, falling back on the wheelchair only when we went to large hospitals, where I pushed her in the wheelchair to speed up the long trips down endless corridors. That day, as we left, Misti pushed the chair herself. As I put the wheelchair in the trunk, it occurred to me that this might be one of the last times I would be doing this chore.

By the time we were in the car and on our way home via the beltway, it was after 5:00 P.M. The traffic was unusually heavy, and I realized that we probably should have had dinner before we left to avoid this traffic. As I mentioned this conversationally to Misti, I was answered by a kick in my side and the remark, "Oh yes, bitch, you can think of that now, but where was your God damned f—-ing mind when you should have thought about it?" Stunned, I watched her foot kick against the windshield, which bent outward. A glance at my rear-view mirror reminded me that getting off the highway at this hour was going to be even harder than trying to control Misti in the moving car. By this time, she was screaming and thrashing her arms and legs, and the almost-forgotten four-letter words started erupting from her mouth.

I had no choice but to keep my attention on the traffic, and by the time I'd gotten off the beltway and onto Route 70, Misti had fallen asleep and stayed asleep until we arrived home about an hour later. Waking up, she was calm and had no recollection of the tantrum in the car. Clearly, though her brain had done much healing, the occasional emotional seizure was still a possibility, especially when she was excited or under stress. It was interesting that this emotional storm had occurred just after an important evaluation during which Misti had been on her best behavior—and just out of range of Dr. Siebens, who was beginning to feel that I was overly concerned about how well Misti could cope.

We began planning the trip to St. Thomas the next day, with the travel agent's assurances that all the hotels and restaurants would be wheelchair accessible. Remembering her own experience recovering from a bad accident, Donna was certainly well-quipped to make this a memorable vacation for Misti. For the first time in years, Misti would be away, separated from us by thousands of miles, with someone close to her own age. We hoped that some time spent in a beautiful place with lots of interesting things to see and do would show Misti that she could function without making so many demands on me.

As I left the travel agency, I asked the agent to make sure the tickets were not on Eastern Airlines, because of rumors of an upcoming strike. I was a bit put off when the agent said, "You must know something we don't." However, I accepted her answer, reasoning that she should certainly be more familiar with this situation than me. She promised to have the tickets to me the day before Misti and Donna were to leave.

The week was a whirl of excitement as Misti and Donna packed and planned. As Donna backed out of the driveway, her little car packed to the roof with the suitcases and wheelchair, I whispered a prayer of thanks and hope to God. Harry and I would celebrate Misti's recovery and our few days of freedom with a trip to Ocean City—a down payment, we hoped, on the many hours we'd be able to spend there relaxing in the future. The days there were wonderfully refreshing, especially after a call from Donna, who reported that the flight had been fine, the hotel was terrific, the weather was lovely, and Misti was having a great time.

Unfortunately, the vicissitudes of life caught up with them a few days later when the rumored strike at Eastern Airlines turned into fact on the very day Misti and Donna were to return home. Donna spent hours standing in long airport lines with Misti in the wheelchair trying to exchange the tickets and being told that no one would honor the tickets of a bankrupt airline. Finally, she called and explained that the only way for them to get home was for her to lay out nearly a thousand dollars for the last two tickets on American. No matter how badly it ended, however, the vacation had done a lot of what we'd hoped for Misti: She had a great time with someone close to her age, and she'd only called us once at the end of the trip when the strike-induced chaos proved overwhelming.

Later that summer, Misti, Harry, and I went back to Baltimore for Misti's driving evaluation, which involved assessing her physical, mental, and emotional abilities. Although Dr. Shapiro had been concerned about Misti's emotional stability when it came to driving, the evaluation went very well—so well that Dr. Siebens said that if he could, he would hand Misti her license back on the spot. Misti was ecstatic. Then, suddenly, out of blue, while we waited in the hallway for Dr. Siebens to do some paperwork, she began screaming, shouting, cursing, kicking, and in general creating an enormous commotion. I had gone down the hall to get a drink of water and was not close, but I saw Dr. Siebens dash out of his office and ask a stunned Harry, "What did you *do* to her?" But Harry had neither said nor done anything to upset her, and he said as much. Dr. Siebens had to admit that based on this display, he agreed with Dr. Shapiro that it wasn't yet safe to give Misti her license back. But, he said to us all, there was nothing to stop him from making another driving license evaluation later as Misti continued to make progress.

By the end of the summer, Misti's continuing progress was obvious and we all (Harry and I, and Drs. Siebens and Shapiro) felt that she was ready to try living on campus. Fortunately, we were able to persuade the administrators at Mont Alto to bend a few rules, and in the fall of 1990, at long last, Misti started living the normal, or nearly normal, life of a dorm resident.

She shared a room with a girl named Sandy, and they shared a bathroom with a third girl. Misti found it difficult to live with her roommate and suite mate. They squabbled over who was messy and who wasn't, who hadn't taken what out of the microwave, as well as facing the usual difficulties of living in tight quarters. But she stuck it out, and she and Sandy became close enough that Sandy joined us all down at Ocean City one weekend over the following summer.

Misti called me a lot that fall—several times a day at first—and she often asked me to come to campus to bring her a sweater or a book she had forgotten at home. Eventually, I had to tell her that I could only speak to her once a day, and so she would have to make sure that she called me about something important. I also made it clear that I was only available to see her on certain specific days because I had to work.

The two of us had fewer conflicts once Misti was living at Mont Alto because she was less dependent on me and thus less angry. The conflicts we did have tended to arise when I tried to point out when her impulses and her behavior were inappropriate and could get her into trouble. As Misti settled into college and dorm life, I frequently took time out from the many happy hours I was spending getting reacquainted with my grandchildren to pray that God would stay with her and keep her safe.

I was especially concerned about the inevitable keg parties because alcohol use is dangerous to anyone who takes Tegretol, making the drug less effective and seizures more likely. Of course, the school authorities did not encourage drinking, but at Mont Alto, as on most college campuses, alcohol was readily available. Misti told me later that since she wanted to socialize with the other kids, she did go to the parties and kept a cup of beer at hand but only took an occasional sip. I fervently hoped that she was really sticking to that strategy; in any case, she did not have seizures, and for that we were grateful.

Misti adjusted well to college life, especially considering the past several years. Still, she clearly lacked insight at times, not only about planning ahead and party behavior, but also about eating properly and her relationships with other people, from roommates to potential boyfriends to classmates and professors. She continued to consult Dr. Shapiro while she was at Mont Alto, however, and she gradually began to moderate some of her responses to people. She tried to persuade us that she was doing just fine, and to a certain degree, she was. She went to class and became part of the crowd, but she also had some sensational quarrels with her roommates. When she got mad, she really got mad, occasionally throwing a humdinger of a tantrum.

After the struggles of the last several years, Harry and I knew that Misti's problematic relationships with other people were not going to improve quickly, regardless of what she might say. Misti still had certain undeniable emotional behavior problems. Drs. Shapiro and Siebens, plus the psychoneurologist we consulted from time to time, all warned that they were certainly not going to go away overnight and might even be with her always.

Of course, now that Misti was away at school and once again in the thick of things, she began interacting with more men. After all, she was an attractive girl, and quite a few fellows were willing to go along with her desire for friendship, if not more. This proved to be a difficult experience for both of us. Even though I knew she still had brain damage and problems in reasoning, I had to learn to let go, to rely on God to watch over her.

Perhaps inevitably, Misti's need for approval and acceptance from her peers resulted in her making some bad choices before she began to accept that many young men saw her as a sexual target. For instance, we had to tell Misti that if she offered to give back rubs to young men on her bed, they would likely think she was coming on to them. I talked to her about this, as did Harry and Dr. Shapiro. We pointed out that though she wasn't ready for a baby at this point, it might happen anyway if she wasn't very careful. We hoped we were getting through to her, but we worried that she might not remember our discussion from one day to the next or would let her guard down at some point. At the very least, though, I suspect that all these chats got Misti to talk about the subject with her roommate Sandy, a friendly and sympathetic girl who was able to give Misti unbiased and reasonable feedback on her behavior.

Often, however, Misti seemed confused, and she would call me. Though her mood seemed to be less erratic as time went on, her insight and ability to reason continued to be more limited than was typical for girls her age. She did make friends, both boys and girls, and it helped that the whole Morningstar family was familiar with the Mont Alto campus. There were plenty of friendly people around who knew Misti and were glad to keep an eye out for her and offer help if necessary. And because the Mont Alto campus was only six miles from Waynesboro, it became common for Misti and her friends to drop in at our place when they wanted to get away from school. Though Misti wasn't yet driving, her friends were, and they were glad to make the trip to Waynesboro for a little home cooking and some TLC from the Morningstars.

Academically, the year was a success. Misti had chosen all of her own classes—since she was becoming more independent all the time, Harry and I were determined to let her make such choices—and she seemed to move naturally toward mathematics and business. However much Misti wanted to fit in by partying with the other kids, she studied enough to end her calculus course with a B-. She did not fare nearly as well in French and English, but did a bit better in economics. Although her plan before the accident had been to concentrate on the hard sciences, she now admitted that science and engineering were too hard and that she could not grasp physics, a subject that she had found quite easy and interesting before the accident.

Misti occasionally complained that the teachers were tough graders, but I suspected these comments really reflected Misti's diminished abilities. Schoolwork was much harder for her than it had ever been before, even though her courses at Mercersburg Academy had been considerably more challenging than many she was taking at Mont Alto.

Gradually, she seemed to take in the fact that she still had some difficulties remaining from the accident, and she also accepted the idea that she'd need some tutoring over the summer if she wanted to keep up her grades in math. She still had great natural ability in the subject, but she needed some review to get to the level she'd need to continue. As time went on, we were able to discuss her inability to concentrate as she once could and her need to study a great deal more than she had before the accident. At the same time that we talked about ways to compensate for her remaining problems, it seemed clear that no amount of studying would bring Misti back to where she'd been before the accident. For instance, math had always been easy for her, but now she confided that she often made simple arithmetic errors that she could not seem to catch even though she checked her work several times. Even so, she continued to insist that she would soon be totally recovered from the brain trauma and go back to being "normal."

When Misti was at Mercersburg Academy, she had never considered going to a community college like Mont Alto, thinking instead of attending Georgetown or Harvard. Now, however, she found herself at a two-year school that granted only associates' degrees, and we had to make plans for her to continue her studies and get her bachelor's degree at another college. Most of her classmates at Mont Alto would be going on to the "main campus"—the large campus of the State University at State College, Pennsylvania. Because her friends would be going on to State College and because the school would automatically accept all of her Mont Alto credits, it was natural for Misti to go there, too. In the fall, then, she would move more than three hours away from Waynesboro, further from home and family than she'd ever been before.

In the meantime, Misti continued to make small adjustments to her new life. Although she was unhappy that she now had to work harder than other students, in general she seemed to become more philosophical, referring to the remainder of her physical problems as "a particularly annoying part of my life." She continued to be plagued with eye problems, such as poor night vision and fatigue, especially when she worked for a long time at the computer. Even years after the accident, she was left with some numbness on the left side of her face, and she limped on her left leg, which she complained felt "numb and funny." She occasionally tripped while walking on campus, and some of her fellow students called her "granny"—not an easy fate for someone who had been a gifted ballerina.

She was embarrassed that her friends had to hang back and walk at a painfully slow pace if they wanted to walk with her. Walking up even a slight hill made her tired and winded; overall, she tired easily and had to nap fairly often. In addition, Misti's short-term memory was still shaky, and she often forgot key matters, such as whether or not she'd already had lunch. As her insight slowly improved, she was able to admit these changes and talk about how depressing they were. Now in daily contact with her peers, she sometimes felt that all of her progress with rehabilitation had stopped, and that was very hard for me to see. I tried to help her see how far she'd come from only the previous year, and I was glad that she'd been able to spend the most difficult days of her recovery at the condo in Ocean City, rather than in Waynesboro, where she'd have constantly been confronted with how much she'd lost and how far she still had to go.

Despite all odds, however, Misti fought off her discouragement and stuck with her schoolwork, studying hard. After her second year at Mont Alto, we went down to Baltimore for another driver's license evaluation, and this time, agreeing with a letter of positive recommendation from Dr. Shapiro, Dr. Siebens certified that Misti was ready to recover her driver's license. She didn't have to take another road test, but for the rest of the summer she and Harry worked on her driving skills, running the family's daily Waynesboro errands together until they both felt she was secure and competent in the car.

By this time, Misti's condition had improved so much that I actually began to look forward to the long trips to doctors' offices because it gave us a chance to talk without interruption. I was especially curious about her views on what had happened just after the accident, and the subject occupied us for many trips and hours of talk. Misti told me that from a very early point, while she was still in the coma, she knew I was there; she could hear me, she said, but didn't understand what I said because I was not speaking a language she understood. Once she had begun to recover slightly, it was her impression that she was in prison, and she could not understand what she had done wrong or why I was keeping her tied up in the carpet-padding warehouse. She told me she recalled a stranger always shaking a silver bell in her face, and that one day, a black man came into her room who helped me load her onto a carpet dolly and put her into the back of a carpet van. She was sure we would take her out into a field and set her free. She had not liked the black man, she said, because he sang like Elvis, and she hated him even more when he helped me take her into the basement of our home, where she was then held prisoner for a long time. She explained that she hated me for doing this to her and that her anger grew because I chased away everyone who came to help her escape.

After one of these trips to Maryland, I would spend hours trying to sort out what she had told me and how it related to her experiences while in coma. I could understand her interpreting her time at Suburban as being in a carpet-padding warehouse. After all, the Morningstar family business was in home furnishings, and she had grown up seeing the six-foot-high rolls of pink, cream, blue, and green carpet padding standing on end. I could well imagine how the tubes in the STU could have reminded her of carpet padding.

The silver bell was a mystery until I went back to Bethesda and came face to face with Nurse Carolyn. Attached to her left shoulder with a large safety pin were the keys to the drug cabinet. It was easy to imagine how someone in a coma could misinterpret the keys as a silver bell hanging in her face as Nurse Carolyn leaned over her to care for her and check the vital machines. The unforgettable character who sang like Elvis was certainly no mystery. It was the young man who had accompanied us in the ambulance on the way to Bryn Mawr Rehab.

As Misti talked to me about her memories, I came to understand how she could be so angry at me, especially since she was forced to be so dependent on me. Since Harry wasn't around on a daily basis, he fell into the category of potential savior rather than target of Misti's rage. I thanked God that we had been blessed with a wonderful doctor like Harvey Shapiro, who could help bring all these things out into the open and help us understand them. Of course, some of Misti's memories of the accident and its aftermath do not pertain to the family at all. I will never forget a conversation that took place on one of our many trips to a doctor's appointment in Baltimore. Riding alone, just the two of us in the car, we talked about her coma, which she referred to as her "long sleep." Curious, I asked her if during that time she ever saw the bright light or long tunnel described by people who have been as close to death as she had been. She put her left hand over on my right leg as I drove, and I could feel the heat from her palm as she replied, "I'm not ready to talk about that yet."

In the fall of 1991, Misti finally went away to school at State College, Pennsylvania. She lived for a year in a dorm, and she enjoyed the life at the school. She declared a major in a demanding course of study, quantitative business analysis—quite an achievement for a girl who had spent months in a deep coma. Still moving slowly at times, and speaking in a slurred voice when she tired, Misti was now able to smile as she explained that "brain trauma is not a disability, just an inconvenience."

For her senior year, Misti wanted to live in an apartment with some other girls, and she did so for a short while. However, she found a place of her own when she got tired of her roommates' rather cruel habits of teasing her about her short-term memory problems. Since she was living on her own with no one nearby to keep track of her, Harry and I made a practice of calling her on the days she didn't call us just to keep in touch and make sure that nothing went wrong. Misti made some friends and went out to movies and football games, but she didn't go out on what she called "date dates," knowing that she needed to use her time to concentrate on her studies.

Then, one weekend, Misti met Rich Lucente, a recent graduate of Penn State who had returned to the campus for homecoming celebrations. A wonderful young man from the Pittsburgh area, Rich was very much taken with Misti's sweetness and beauty. Although Misti teased that Harry and I liked Rich because he was a "nerd"—her word for nonjocks whose approach to college involved hard work and getting good grades—it was clear that she liked him, too.

In early spring of Misti's senior year, Rich took a Thursday off work and drove to State College. Carrying a dozen red roses, he walked into Misti's math class and up the aisle to her desk. There, he dropped to his knees and in front of a full room of interested classmates put the roses in her lap, pulled a sparkling oval diamond from his pocket, looked into her eyes, and proposed to her. "I love you, Misti and want to spend the rest of my life with you. Will you marry me?" The class clapped and cheered, "Say yes, Misti, say yes!" And she did.

As we planned and prepared for the wedding, I was haunted by a feeling that I could not shake. Even though I tried to explain about Misti's sometimes difficult behavior and showed him some of the videos that had been taken at Bryn Mawr, I was not completely sure that Rich could fully comprehend the problems that brain trauma can leave in its wake. I knew that marriage is not always a smooth road, and I feared that this one would be rockier than most, given Misti's still erratic moods and strong reactions to people. Though they say that love conquers all, I had seen at the Rehab that there are problems that even the deepest love cannot conquer. I felt as though I was handing Rich my responsibility and hoped that he would be able to handle whatever might face him in the future. And I prayed.

☙

On July 17, 1993, a few weeks after Misti graduated from Penn State University and five years, five months, and fifteen days after the accident, the bells in the carillons of Mercersburg Academy rang out. Misti appeared at the rear of the Mercersburg Academy Chapel, a vision in white, trailing yards of white satin, pearls, and lace. Using only her father's arm for support, she walked down the hundred-foot flagstone aisle to unite with her true love.

Larry Jones, Mercersburg's one-time chaplain and Misti's good friend, had done the premarriage counseling for Misti and Rich. Now he opened the wedding service before some three hundred friends and relatives with the words, "Today, we gather here to witness a miracle." Tears flowed from his eyes and from those of many in the assembled congregation—tears of joy, tears of gratitude, and for many, tears of hope rewarded and doubts swept away.

The next day, before packing away the journals that I had been keeping since the accident, I inserted a card that Misti had sent me the previous October for my birthday. Selected with great care and mailed from State College, it read, "To my best friend—Happy Birthday. I know this is mushy, but I really mean it. Love, Misti."

Harry and I then sat down and talked, mostly about the finances of the wedding. Were all the bills paid? Had the fee for the flowers been taken care of? Had we perhaps forgotten some expense that would crop up later? I assured Harry that everything for the wedding had been taken care of, and he replied that even if we put a little money aside for some completely forgotten wedding bill, we would still have money left to buy the sixteen-foot Boston Whaler he had been longing for. A few days later, we took off to Washington, D.C. and picked up the boat at the boatyard. As we drove down Route 50 to Ocean City, he looked at me with a smile and said that now we were starting our perpetual vacation. For the first time in many years, we were together and without major responsibilities. Older, but wiser, we were ready to start our new life together—the life we had thought we were starting over five years before.

EPILOGUE

On May 14, 1996, Misti and Rich were blessed with a son, Christian Ray.

Now that Misti is launched into life, I am able to look back on this very hard time in our lives, and I realize that Misti is not the only one who has changed. I've changed, too. I learned some tough and valuable lessons. Some are medical: I've been through rehabilitation of a loved one after traumatic brain injury, and I know what it entails. In the years since Misti's accident, I've been able to give comfort and hope to other parents whose children have been injured, and I've been glad to do so. I've seen what can happen to the brain, and I've seen what can't be fixed. On the other hand, I know that recovery is possible, even under difficult circumstances. I think back now to what the doctors at Suburban told us about Misti right after the accident—that she might not live and if she lived, she would be so damaged that we would not recognize her as a person. We were told that the brain heals for only about eighteen months after injury and that after that time there could be no more recovery. Well, statistically, the doctors and oddsmakers may be right, but Misti's progress demonstrates that sometimes, when one is lucky and when there is a will to do better, recovery can go on for years.

I've also learned a lot about the unpredictability and fragility of human life. Before Misti's accident, if I saw someone who was handicapped, I saw the handicap before the person; now if I see someone in a wheelchair, I'm very aware of the person and consciously take the time to help if it's needed and to give a kind word. That person could be anyone of us—me, you, your daughter or son.

I'm not the person I was before the accident. Now I speak up early if something seems wrong, and I make sure that things get taken care of properly. I've done things I never thought I'd be able to do, from standing up for myself and my daughter to driving the beltway. Those

191

were unlooked-for pluses in a bad situation. On the other hand, I've never gotten back the same sense of concentration I had before the accident.

I've become both more and less patient since then: I have a hard time listening to people who go on and on about minor problems or take a "poor me" stance to their lives, and I don't have much patience with anyone who is lazy or plays Hamlet while making decisions. At the same time, I take—and make—much more time for what's really important: my family, especially my grandchildren, beauty, and good friends.

☺

Often, as a teenager and young woman, I wondered why I was alive, what I had been put on earth to do.

When I married, I knew it was not just to be a wife and helpmate to Harry. I loved being a mother, and I was good at it, but even though it was a very important job, one that tested me in many ways, I knew it was not the answer to the questions in my mind. Nor did several decades as a successful decorator fill my need for more. Though my career was satisfying, it only made me more certain that I had not yet found the job that God had in mind for me.

But now, looking at Misti and her lovely family and praying for their success in meeting the challenges of the years ahead, I finally feel that I know what I was born to do.

As I watch Misti move through life facing not only the ups and downs that most people do but also dealing with the continuing aftermath of brain injury, I thank God that he gave me the drive to carry on the task he assigned me. Almost like a minister feeling the call to serve, I can look back now and see how my life prepared me to do what I had been called to do. I consider my parents, who taught me the importance of hard work and faith; the teachers and ministers who reinforced Mommie and Daddy's teachings; the many family members who were part of my early life; the contributions of Harry and Chuck and Cork; my coworkers, friends, and many more.

I marvel at how fate dealt the cards to total strangers who sired and conceived a child that they found impossible to abort and how they chose instead to entrust her life to us. Even though they will never know it, by making their sacrifices, Misti's birth parents were responsible for me completing my life's challenge. And she was blessed with wonderful guardian angels along the way: Mrs. Broadwater, Nurses Carolyn and Peggy, Cathy Cosgrove, Kay Yaukey, Donna Kaufman.

It always amazes me how the events in our lives, no matter how insignificant, build one upon the other to complete the great tapestry of our lives and how we may never know the impact of each until the plan is finally completed.

Time will never erase the memories of the difficulties we had to endure. And there is no guarantee of continued progress, for brain injury can be cruel and capricious in its results. In some ways, Misti will continue to struggle with the effects of the accident for her whole life, as will those who love her. But nothing can ever take away what we have accomplished.